"Will we ever really understand that state of mind and decade we call "the sixties"? It left permanent marks on our society including changes in psychology, politics, the food we eat, how we think about mental and physical health, and much more. Lattin has crafted a riveting account of four of the personalities who deeply influenced those cultural shifts. . . for good or for ill. A skillfully woven group biography, it is thoroughly researched, wonderfully readable, and sparkles with keen insights. Tim Leary, Richard Alpert (Ram Dass), Andrew Weil, and Huston Smith all come alive, both as fascinating personalities and in their intricate relationships with each other. This is not just a book about magic mushrooms or LSD. It is the story of a turning point we are still living with."

— Harvey Cox, Hollis Research Professor of Divinity, Harvard University, author of *The Future of Faith*

"A revealing account of four iconic personalities who helped define an era, sowed seeds of consciousness, and left indelible marks in the lives of spiritual explorers to this day. The conclusion alone is worth the price of the book."

— Dan Millman, author of *The Peaceful Warrior*

"This book is a real trip, as we used to say, and it will probably give you flashbacks whether you were there or not. Lattin does a grand job of telling us the wildly improbable story of psychedelic drugs in America, and the jump start of the "new age" spiritual movement. A very far-out read!"

— Wes "Scoop" Nisker, author, Buddhist meditation teacher, and performer

# The HARVARD PSYCHEDELIC CLUB

Also by Don Lattin:

*JESUS FREAKS: A True Story of Murder and Madness on the Evangelical Edge*

*FOLLOWING OUR BLISS: How the Spiritual Ideals of the Sixties Shape Our Lives Today*

*SHOPPING FOR FAITH: American Religion in the New Millennium* (with Richard Cimino)

# The HARVARD PSYCHEDELIC CLUB

*How Timothy Leary, Ram Dass,
Huston Smith, and Andrew Weil
Killed the Fifties and
Ushered in a New Age for America*

## Don Lattin

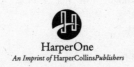

HarperOne
*An Imprint of HarperCollinsPublishers*

HarperOne

Grateful acknowledgement is made to reprint the interview with Timothy Leary on pages 120–121 that was originally published in *Playboy* magazine in September 1966.

HarperCollins books may be purchased for educational, business, or sales promotional use. For information please write: Special Markets Department, HarperCollins Publishers, 10 East 53rd Street, New York, NY 10022.

HarperCollins Web site: http://www.harpercollins.com

HarperCollins®, 🏭®, and HarperOne™ are trademarks of HarperCollins Publishers

FIRST EDITION

Library of Congress Cataloging-in-Publication Data is available upon request.

ISBN 978–0–06–165593–7

10 11 12 13 14 RRD(H) 10 9 8 7 6 5 4 3 2 1

To Paul and Cheryl

# CONTENTS

CHAPTER ONE

## Four Roads to Cambridge    5

*Huston Smith (born in Soochow, China, in 1919), Timothy Leary
(born in Springfield, Massachusetts, in 1920), Richard Alpert
(born in Boston, Massachusetts, in 1931), and Andrew Weil
(born in Philadelphia, Pennsylvania, in 1942) find their
way to Harvard and cross paths in the fall of 1960.*

CHAPTER TWO

## Turn On    37

*Between the summer of 1960 and the winter of 1961,
the founding fathers of the Harvard Psychedelic Club
get their first taste of the "flesh of the gods." Cameo
appearances by Aldous Huxley and Allen Ginsberg.*

CHAPTER THREE

## Sinners and Saints    61

*Leary, Smith, and an inspired band of graduate students begin their
first two research projects, giving psychedelic drugs to convicts at
Concord Prison in the spring of 1961 and, one year later, to seminary
students attending a worship service on Good Friday. Cameo
appearance by Bill Wilson, the founder of Alcoholics Anonymous.*

CHAPTER FOUR

## Crimson Tide    85

*Leary and Alpert deny Andrew Weil membership into the
Harvard Psychedelic Club, saying they are not allowed to include
undergraduate students. Weil gets jealous when Alpert starts
courting one of his friends and initiates that undergraduate
into the psychedelic fold. Then Andrew gets his revenge with
a damning exposé published in the Harvard Crimson.*

CHAPTER FIVE

## Trouble in Paradise    107

*Weil's article gets Leary and Alpert kicked out of Harvard in the
spring of 1963, turning them into media celebrities and national
spokesmen for a generation turning to LSD for instant enlightenment.
Huston Smith decides drugs are not the answer. Leary and Alpert
have a falling-out over Alpert's infatuation with young men.*

CHAPTER SIX

## If You Come to San Francisco . . .    119

*By 1966, the San Francisco Bay area has become the
center of the psychedelic cyclone. Leary, Smith, Weil, and
Alpert—along with countless other seekers—go west to
check out the scene. Cameo appearances by Ken Kesey,
John Lennon, Grace Slick, and Jerry Garcia.*

CHAPTER SEVEN

## Pilgrimage and Exile    149

*Smith seeks enlightenment in Japan, Weil follows the flesh
of the gods into South America, and Alpert travels to India,
returning as Ram Dass. Meanwhile, Leary gets tossed in jail,
escapes with the help of the Weather Underground, and then
goes into exile in Algeria, Switzerland, and Afghanistan.*

CHAPTER EIGHT

## After the Ecstasy . . . Four Lives 181

*There's a lesson to be learned in the various ways that Leary,*
*Alpert, Weil, and Smith took the psychedelic experience*
*and incorporated it into the rest of their lives.*

CONCLUSION

## Healer, Teacher, Trickster, Seeker 211

*How did the life work of Andrew Weil, Huston Smith, Timothy Leary,*
*and Richard Alpert transform the way we live our lives today?*

# ILLUSTRATIONS

## AUTHOR'S NOTE

This is a work of narrative nonfiction. The dialogue in this book is the author's rendition of what was actually said in these conversations. It is based on interviews with the speakers, written accounts from those involved, and other research into the various characters' state of mind. When possible, the re-created dialogue was reviewed by at least one of the participants in a conversation. For more information on the sources used to re-create various scenes, please refer to "Notes on Source Material" at the end of the book.

# Introduction

This book is the story of three brilliant scholars and one ambitious freshman who crossed paths at Harvard University in the winter of 1960–61, and how their experiences in a psychedelic drug research project transformed their lives and much of American culture in the 1960s and 1970s. It's about the intersecting life stories of Timothy Leary, a research psychologist and proponent of enlightenment through LSD; Huston Smith, an MIT philosophy professor and widely read expert on the world's religions; Richard Alpert, a Harvard psychology professor who traveled to India and returned as Ram Dass; and Dr. Andrew Weil, a Harvard Medical School graduate who became the nation's best-known proponent of holistic health and natural foods.

They came together at an extraordinary time and place in American history. It was the end of the 1950s—a decade defined by conformity, consumerism, political paranoia, and the just-discovered nightmare of global nuclear annihilation. It was the beginning of the 1960s, which would see its own horrors and divisive politics but was somehow redeemed by a new spirit of optimism, innovation, and hope. Massachusetts senator John F. Kennedy, a Harvard graduate, had just been elected president of the United States, making him the youngest man to ever hold that office. Kennedy put together a cabinet by cherry-picking Harvard's best and brightest.

Was there a reason these four men came together at this time and place? Perhaps it's just a coincidence, but some extraordinary spirit rose out of Harvard in the fall of 1960. *Something's happening here. What it is ain't exactly clear.* Timothy Leary discovers the wondrous world of magic mushrooms during his summer break in Mexico, just as seventeen-year-old Andrew Weil is getting ready to come to Harvard to study botany. Aldous Huxley, the great British novelist and student of human consciousness, just happens to be lecturing that fall at nearby MIT. Huxley hears about Leary, then introduces Leary to his old friend Huston Smith. Allen Ginsberg, the Beat poet who seems to pop up everywhere in the fifties, sixties, and seventies, is crashing at Leary's house that fall. One of Leary's colleagues in the Harvard psychology department, Richard Alpert, is, when the merriment begins, on loan to the University of California at Berkeley, but he lays the groundwork for a psychedelic drug culture that is about to burst forth in Boston, San Francisco, and, from there, around the world.

They came together at a time of upheaval and experimentation, and they set the stage for the social, spiritual, sexual, and psychological revolution of the 1960s. Smith would be The Teacher, educating three generations to adopt a more tolerant, inclusive attitude toward other people's religions. Alpert would be The Seeker, inspiring a restless army of spiritual pilgrims. Weil would be The Healer, devoting his life to the holistic reformation of the American health-care system. And Leary would play The Trickster, advising a generation to "turn on, tune in, and drop out."

They would help define the decade, so much so that John Lennon would write two Beatles songs for their story's soundtrack—"Tomorrow Never Knows," about his Leary-inspired acid trip, and "Come Together," originally conceived as a campaign song for The Trickster's whimsical race against Ronald Reagan for governor of California. *One thing I can tell you is you got to be free.* Other tunes would be cut by the Jefferson Airplane, the Grateful Dead, and the Moody Blues, whose song "The Legend of a Mind" would let us know whether Timothy Leary was dead, or just *on the outside, looking in.*

They came together, then drifted apart, but the cultural changes they wrought are still very much with us today. There would be a time of joy, a time of peace, and a time of love. There would also be times of backstabbing, jealousy, and outright betrayal. *A time to dance. A time to mourn.* And it would take Richard Alpert more than one lifetime to forgive Andrew Weil for what he did to him and his career back at the dawning of the Age of Aquarius.

Leary would go on to become one of the most revered and reviled symbols of the 1960s. Huston Smith would enthusiastically join Leary's psychedelic crusade, only to go his own way when the party got a little wild for an ordained, and happily married, Methodist minister. Richard Alpert, as Ram Dass, would continue to struggle with a voracious omni-sexual appetite. Andy Weil would play hardball in his campaign to get Alpert and Leary kicked out of Harvard, only to replace them in the 1970s as the new ringmaster of the drug culture.

Smith, Leary, Alpert, and Weil were all career-driven, linear-thinking intellectuals before their consciousness-expanding encounters with psilocybin mushrooms, LSD, and other psychedelic drugs. After the ecstasy, they all turned from intellect to intuition, from mechanistic thinking to mysticism, from the scholarly to the spiritual, from the scientific to the shamanic. The men of the Harvard Psychedelic Club, each in his own way, changed the way Americans think, practice medicine, and view religion; that is, they changed nothing less than the way we look at mind, body, and spirit.

# CHAPTER ONE

# Four Roads to Cambridge

## Seeker
## Cambridge, Massachusetts
## Spring 1961

Richard Alpert, an assistant professor in clinical psychology at Harvard University, was on track. Tenure track. Alpert was still in his twenties, but he already had the big corner office in the Department of Social Relations. He had twin appointments in psychology and education. His private life seemed just as sweet. His Cambridge apartment was filled with exquisite antiques. He had a Mercedes sedan, an MG sports car, a Triumph motorcycle, and his own Cessna airplane. It was the dawn of the swinging sixties, and Alpert was all set for life in the fast lane. What made it even sweeter was that none of this was supposed to happen. He'd shown those bastards. Here he was, teaching at Harvard—a place that wouldn't even accept him as a student, even *with* all of his father's New England connections.

Just nine years ago, he'd nearly flunked out of college and seemed destined to fail at the profession his father had chosen for him—medical doctor. But that time, Richard was the one thumbing his nose at daddy's connections. That was back in the spring of 1952, just before he got his undergraduate degree from Tufts University. One day in his senior year, Tufts president Leonard Carmichael called Alpert to his office.

"So, Richard," he said. "I understand you want to be a psychologist."

Alpert thought Carmichael, himself an eminent psychologist, was about to congratulate him on his career choice.

"Yes, sir," Richard replied. "I want to be a social psychologist."

"You'd make a terrible psychologist. How about going to medical school?"

"I don't want to go to medical school."

"You know, Richard, your father really wants you to go to medical school. Tufts has a fine medical school."

"I know it does, and I know my father wants me to go to medical school. We're Jewish. He's a lawyer. I'm supposed to be a doctor or a lawyer. But I don't want to go to medical school. My grades in my premed courses were awful. I want to be a psychologist."

"Just a minute, Richard."

President Carmichael picked up the phone and called the head of the Tufts University School of Medicine.

"Hey. I've got George Alpert's son in my office over here. Bright kid. You got a space for him over there? This is a personal favor."

"That's great. . . . Thanks much," Carmichael said, hanging up the phone.

"Congratulations, son. You're in medical school."

"President Carmichael, I wouldn't go to medical school if you paid me," the thankless student replied. "I'm going into psychology."

George Alpert found out about the conversation, and he was furious. Richard was the youngest of his three sons, born on April 6, 1931, before his family joined the white flight out of Roxbury and moved to the safer streets of Newton, Massachusetts. George wasn't worried about his other boys, who were five and ten years older than little Richard. They'd be fine. William, the oldest, had been a great athlete; Leonard, his other brother, was a great musician. But Dick was different. He was a cute little boy, the Tinker Bell of the family. He seemed to be a happy child, but he really wasn't that happy—especially after his parents sent him to Williston Academy in Easthampton, Massachusetts, the prep school that had done such a fine job preparing his older brothers for their academic careers.

Things started off all right for Richard at Williston, where he worked on the school newspaper and excelled at tennis. But in his early teens, he started having strange feelings about some of the other boys at school. Sexual feelings. One day, a few classmates caught Richard wrestling in the nude with another student. Word soon spread around Williston that Dickie Alpert was queer. His classmates started the silent treatment—ignoring him whenever he'd walk into a room. Richard knew they were right. He hated to admit it, but he *was* queer.

His homosexuality was something to hide, and for the most part, during college and during his time at Harvard, that's exactly what he did. Even in the 1960s and 1970s, when Alpert was famous and it was safer to say you were gay, he kept silent about his sexuality.

It wasn't reported at the time, but his romantic attraction to undergraduate men was one of the sins that would get him kicked out of Harvard in the spring of 1963. It would also spark a long estrangement from Timothy Leary, who would go so far as to condemn his colleague's sexual orientation as "evil." Alpert doesn't mention it in an otherwise revealing autobiographical chapter in *Be Here Now,* the spiritual classic that was published in 1971 and put him on the counterculture map, but his sexual frustrations were one of the reasons he went off to India, from which he returned, reincarnated, as Ram Dass.

Back at Tufts in the 1950s, Alpert learned how to hide his homosexuality. He refined those skills at Wesleyan University in Middletown, Connecticut, where he struggled academically but left with a master's degree in psychology. The chairman of the psychology department at Wesleyan, David McClelland, liked Alpert and used his connections to get Richard into the doctoral program at Stanford University. Once again, Alpert fell behind in his studies and was nearly thrown out of school. About to lose his scholarship, and terrified at the prospect of having to tell his father about his failure, Richard started studying all night long. He somehow managed to improve his grades and get his doctoral degree from Stanford, then land a teaching job there fresh out of school. Young Alpert's charm and charisma concealed whatever failings he had as a scholar and researcher. He was a fantastic lecturer—a favorite among undergraduates. That's what got him the Stanford job.

It seemed like a perfect fit as Alpert settled into his new life in Palo Alto, a town just south of San Francisco. He was teaching Stanford undergraduates and working as a psychotherapist at the university health clinic. His first therapy patient there was Vik Lovell, a graduate student who would soon turn Alpert on to marijuana. In a few years, the writer Ken Kesey would dedicate *One Flew Over the Cuckoo's Nest* to Lovell, calling him the man "who told me dragons did not exist, then led me to their lairs." This was several years before Alpert and Kesey would be introduced to psychedelics in disparate scenes on the East and West coasts. Lovell would have the distinction of being the guy who first told Kesey about the amazing effects LSD had on the human mind. Kesey would later form the Merry Pranksters, a guerrilla theater group that would stage a series of "Acid Tests" around the San Francisco Bay area, public events featuring light shows, the Grateful Dead, and a free-flowing supply of psychedelic drugs.

Lovell was also Alpert's first introduction to the budding social network that would soon blossom into the sixties counterculture. But that was still a few years off. At the time, the young professor-therapist was shocked and a bit disgusted when Lovell walked into Alpert's Stanford office and swung his dirty feet up onto the therapist's desk. Alpert had seen some of this student's rather licentious writing, and was even a bit shocked by the guy's dirty mind. Now this guy had the gall to walk into Alpert's office, lift his feet onto his desk, and push the professor's potted plant out of his way to make himself a bit more comfortable.

Five years later, when Alpert had become an infamous proponent of LSD, Alpert and Lovell had another meeting. Alpert was visiting the Bay Area, lecturing on drugs and hanging out with some members of the Hells Angels. One of the bikers loaned Alpert his Harley for the afternoon, and Richard headed down Pacific Coast Highway to visit some of his old Stanford haunts. When he walked into his old office, whom did he find there but Vik Lovell, sitting at his old desk and performing his old job at the student clinic. Alpert walked into the office, tore open his leather jacket, sat down, and swung his dirty boots up on the desk. They both laughed so hard they practically fell out of their chairs. Then they went out for a beer.

A lot can happen in five years, and that was certainly the case in Richard Alpert's life between 1958 and 1963. David McClelland, who had been Alpert's mentor at Wesleyan and helped him get the Stanford job, had been hired by Harvard to direct the university's new Center for Personality Research. He offered Alpert a job. Suddenly, the struggling grad student and closeted homosexual had dueling offers from two of the nation's most prestigious universities. Being a Boston boy, Alpert took the Harvard job.

In the late 1950s, Alpert was working at Harvard and finishing up a research project at Stanford. By this time, Alpert had almost gotten used to dividing his life between an East Coast and West Coast existence. It began when he was still a struggling student at Stanford. By that time, his father had become president of the New Haven Railroad and was trying to bring his wayward son into the rail business. Richard reluctantly agreed to spend a few days a month back in New York helping dad out with the company. In those days it took fourteen hours to fly from San Francisco to New York. At Stanford, Alpert was running the coffee lounge in the psychology department, collecting spare change to make sure there were enough cups for the other graduate students. In New York, he would be met at the airport by a chauffeured limousine and whisked to an office where he'd help his father decide what kind of locomotives they should buy. He kept his life as a New York businessman a secret from his Stanford pals, who wouldn't think that was a very cool scene. Back in the Bay Area, Alpert had taken on the role of a hip college professor, smoking pot at parties and trying to look wise. His friends started calling him "The Shrink," and Richard played the part well.

But there were other, deeper secrets. At one point, Alpert was simultaneously living with a male lover in San Francisco and a female partner in Boston. Neither the boyfriend nor the girlfriend knew anything about the other lover. Dick wasn't even sure if he was gay or straight. All he knew was that he was living a lie. He was living the ultimate life, but he was living a lie.

In the summer of 1959, one of Alpert's Harvard students, an undergraduate named Jim Fadiman, got an intimate view of his professor's bisexual, bicoastal existence. Alpert offered Jim a job as a summer research assistant to help out on his Stanford research— a study of mathematical learning skills among elementary school kids. Alpert and Fadiman wound up living together in a house in Palo Alto that Alpert had rented from a Stanford professor who was away for the summer. They had a great time working and hanging out together, and soon settled into a routine. They'd finish up a day of research, then go buy some food and head home to prepare the evening meal. Fadiman would later wonder if Alpert saw him as a potential lover, but at the time, the twenty-year-old was an extremely innocent young man. In fact, he was still a virgin. Fadiman didn't think of himself as heterosexual or homosexual. He wasn't sexual at all. But his roommate certainly seemed to be interested in all of the above.

Despite his inexperience in sexual matters, Fadiman was able to offer some insight into Alpert's love life.

They were having breakfast one morning. Alpert was back from one of his many dates. Jim moved the scrambled eggs around on his plate, gathering up the courage to offer an observation.

"Hey, Dick, can I tell you something?" Jim asked.

"Of course," Richard replied. "You can tell me anything."

"Well, I've noticed that the women you are sleeping with this summer seem to be a lot brighter than the men you are sleeping with," Jim said. "The women seem to be bright, capable women. The men just seem pretty."

Alpert took a sip of coffee and looked up at the wise undergraduate. "Yeah," he said. "I guess that's true."

Their friendship continued during Fadiman's senior year back at Harvard. One night that year, Alpert took him to a gay bar in Boston. It was a revelation to Fadiman that such a place even existed. And while there may have been some sexual signals, Jim never picked them up, and the professor never made a real pass. At Harvard, Alpert pretended he was straight, while out in San Francisco, the gay side seemed to flower.

Jim noticed a few other things about his favorite professor. While Alpert was supposedly the mentor in their relationship, he would show flashes of insecurity about his own intellectual abilities. This insecurity was actually one of Alpert's more charming characteristics, and it would express itself as Professor Richard Alpert, and in his later incarnation as Ram Dass. In both roles, Alpert made a career out of this charismatic mix of personal insight, bemused self-deprecation, and true confession. It made people love him, and Richard loved to be loved.

One night, Fadiman and Alpert went out to see a production of Samuel Beckett's existential comedy *Waiting for Godot,* a play that Fadiman—not Alpert—wanted to see. As they were walking to the theater, the professor turned to the student and quipped, "If this is one of those plays where afterward I'm going to say, 'I didn't understand a thing,' and you're going to look down on me, then I don't want to go." Of course, it *was* one of those plays. Alpert wasn't sure *what* it was about. Fadiman didn't really get it, either, but he tried his best to make it seem as if he did.*

---

*Fadiman would reappear in a later chapter of psychedelic history. In his book *What the Dormouse Said: How the Sixties Counterculture Shaped the Personal Computer Industry,* John Markoff shows how key Silicon Valley pioneers, including Apple cofounder Steve Jobs, and Douglas Engelbart, the man who invented the mouse, were inspired, in part, by their psychedelic experiences. Engelbart was turned on by Fadiman after Alpert's former student went on to do LSD

To most people, including Fadiman, Richard seemed fairly content with his life. But Alpert would later see these years as a time of alienation and hidden depression. "In the face of this feeling of malaise, I ate more, collected more possessions, collected more appointments and positions and status, more sexual and alcoholic orgies, and more wildness in my life. Every time I went to a family gathering, I was the boy who made it. I was the professor at Harvard and everybody stood around in awe and listened to my every word, and all I felt was the horror that I knew inside that I didn't know. Of course, it was all such beautiful, gentle horror, because there was so much reward involved."

It was David McClelland, his old mentor at Wesleyan, who got him the Harvard job. McClelland had moved up the academic ladder and had brought his bright young protégé along. Alpert was given a huge corner office in an old mansion that housed the Center for Personality Research, which was part of Harvard's Department of Social Relations. One afternoon in the fall of 1959, McClelland walked into that office. He'd just come back from a sabbatical in Europe and had some big news.

"When I was in Europe," McClelland said, "I came across this interesting psychologist who is bright as hell. He was there bicycling across Italy or something. Anyway, I offered him a job. Do you have any idea where we can put him?"

"Well," Alpert replied, "there's a broom closet down the hall. We can put him there."

---

research in the early 1960s at the International Foundation for Advanced Study in Menlo Park, California, looking at how psychedelic drugs can foster creativity. Another psychedelic pioneer to emerge as a Silicon Valley trailblazer was Stewart Brand, one of Ken Kesey's original Merry Pranksters. Brand, an early personal-computing enthusiast and Internet pioneer, went on to found the *Whole Earth Catalog,* a back-to-the-land, hippie-inspired version of the Sears Roebuck catalogue. "The counterculture's scorn for centralized authority," he argues, "provided the philosophical foundations of not only the leaderless Internet but also the entire personal-computer revolution."

"Oh, by the way, his name's Leary," McClelland said. "Tim Leary."

Trickster
Berkeley, California
Fall 1955

---

On the morning of his thirty-fifth birthday, Timothy Leary woke up in his home in the Berkeley hills and found a note on his wife's pillow. "What now?" Leary asked himself. "More drama?" They'd had another martini-fueled fight the night before, the main issue being Leary's latest infidelity. It wasn't so much that Leary was being unfaithful. He and his wife, Marianne, had what would later be called an "open relationship." They called it "wife swapping" back in the fifties. Tim and Marianne both liked to flirt. The martini parties they held at their home at 1230 Queens Road had become notorious among the clinical psychologists down the hill on the University of California campus. Leary loved to hold court in his spacious home, which offered sweeping views of San Francisco Bay. He loved keeping the gin chilled, making sure the glasses were filled, and speculating as to which guests were on the verge of pairing up.

In recent weeks, Marianne had been becoming increasingly depressed about their marriage. Little flings were OK. Marianne was having one of them herself at the time with a married man. "They had a deal," a friend explained. "They would always stay together. The deal was that they just couldn't fall in love with their lovers. They could fuck around, but they couldn't fall in love." Tim was breaking the deal. Marianne was sure he was about to run off with his lover and leave her and their two children—Susan, who was eight years old, and Jack, who was five. Marianne was right in her suspicions. Tim was getting seriously involved with his latest lover. He'd even rented a little apartment down on Telegraph Avenue where they'd meet up several times a week for their liaisons. Marianne was downing tranquilizers and drinking heavily. She was fed up with the state of their marriage, but at the same time desperately wanted to save it.

Tim woke up on his birthday morning with a vague recollection of the previous night's dispute. "I can't go on like this!" his wife had screamed.

"That's your problem," he replied, then retired for the evening.

In the morning, Leary reached over and unfolded the note on the pillow.

"My darling," it read. "I cannot live without your love. I have loved life, but through you. The children will grow up wondering about their mother. I love them so much and please tell them that. Please be good to them. They are so dear."

Leary bolted out of bed. He could hear the car running. Shouting his wife's name, he ran into the garage. Choking on exhaust fumes, he swung open the door. Marianne was lying across the front seat in her nightgown. The kids heard all the commotion and ran out in their pajamas. "Susan! Run down to the firehouse," Leary said. "Tell them to bring oxygen!"

Tim hopped into the ambulance for the ride down the hill to Herrick Memorial Hospital, but it was too late. Marianne Busch Leary, thirty-three, was pronounced dead at 9:28 A.M. The Alameda County Coroner's Office listed the death as a "probable suicide."

In his autobiography, published three decades and four wives later, Leary would single out one mind-altering drug—alcohol— as the cause of a series of tragedies that would haunt at least three generations of the Leary family. "Booze ruined my father's life, smashed his marriage, eroded the lives of four uncles. Marianne's suicide and thus the endless sorrows of my children were due to booze."

Those sorrows continued after the 1983 publication of Tim's memoir, *Flashbacks*. Seven years later, in 1990, Susan Leary would hang herself in a jail cell while awaiting trial for attempted murder. Jack Leary, who would have his own troubles with the law, would become estranged from his father in the 1970s. They would never really reconcile before Timothy Leary's death at his Los Angeles home on May 31, 1996.

Timothy Leary was born in Springfield, Massachusetts, on October 22, 1920. He liked to say that he was conceived the day after Prohibition was enacted in the United States. His life began, in utero, on the night of January 27, 1920. His father, a dentist and a captain in the U.S. Army at West Point, didn't let the new law against alcohol get in the way of his drinking.

World War I was still raging across Europe when Timothy Leary Sr. married Abigail Ferris on January 7, 1918, just months after he was commissioned into the Army Dental Corps. That post allowed Tote, as he was known, to avoid seeing action in the Great War. It also provided an opportunity after the war for him to hobnob with such luminaries as General Douglas MacArthur, Captain Omar Bradley, and Lieutenant George Patton.

During her pregnancy, Abigail Leary was sometimes overcome by the sour smell of bathtub gin that hung over the officers' quarters like "rowdy smog." But the years following the war were the high point of the otherwise unremarkable life of Captain Leary, who soon returned to Springfield and set up a small dental practice.

Young Timothy's earliest memories of life with father revolve around Dad coming home late at night—drunk and disorderly. One night, when Tim was twelve years old, he got up the courage to yell down the stairs, "Hey! We're trying to sleep up here!"

Tote responded with rage. "I'll teach you a thing or two right now," he yelled, climbing up toward his son.

Tim looked into the threatening face, and when his father got to the top of the stairs, he pushed him back, causing him to tumble back down the stairway, head over heels. Tote crashed into a telephone stand, busted his glasses, but managed to right himself and head back up the stairs, screaming, "I'll get you for that."

As he had many times before, Tim jumped out of an upstairs window, ran up a steep gabled roof, and climbed back down a drainpipe, hiding behind the chimney until his mother let him know that his father had passed out and it was safe to come back inside.

His father's alcoholism only worsened, causing Tote to lose his dental practice, disappear from Springfield, and abandon his family in the midst of the Great Depression. Life lurched on for the Leary clan, and—despite a reputation for skipping school more than any other student in his senior class—Timothy graduated from Springfield's Classical High School in June 1938.

Leary, like Alpert, didn't have the grades to get into an Ivy League school, so at his mother's urging Tim went off for a Jesuit education at the College of the Holy Cross in nearby Worcester. Despite mediocre grades in his sophomore year, young Leary managed to fulfill another of his mother's dreams and transfer to West Point in the fall of 1940. But Leary had a rebellious streak that seemed destined to get him kicked out of the elite officer-training academy. His troubles began when he got so drunk following the Army–Navy football game in December 1940 that he was unable to stand up the next day at morning reveille. Leary was asked to resign from the academy, but he refused and was subjected to Coventry, or "silencing"—a disciplinary practice in which his fellow cadets were forbidden to talk with him or socialize in any way. Leary was undergoing this banishment around the same time that Alpert (who was eleven years younger than Tim) had been labeled "queer" and was getting the silent treatment from his classmates at Williston Academy.

Leary's tough times at West Point had a lasting effect on his philosophy of life. "I have changed so much," he wrote in a letter to his mother. "I am so scared of the world at times and then I feel that after all it makes no difference what becomes of me, that I shall always be happy because I will not take myself too seriously. This is one of my new philosophies and it is the thing that keeps me from minding the men around here who silence me."

Tim managed to hang on at West Point and leave the army with an honorable discharge in September 1941—just three months before the bombing of Pearl Harbor brought the United States into World War II. Leary's odyssey for an undergraduate degree took him to the University of Alabama, where he avoided active service by enrolling in the ROTC. That made him eligible for a special program that offered psychology majors three months of study at Georgetown University and six months at Ohio State. Following those studies, he managed to sit out the rest of the war as a psychometrician, a measurer of mental traits, at Deshon General Hospital in Butler, Pennsylvania, where he began his ill-fated courtship with Marianne Busch.

Marianne grew up in a suburb of Portland, Oregon. Her roots in the Pacific Northwest were what originally inspired the young married couple to head out to the West Coast, first to Washington State University, where Tim got his master's degree in psychology, and then to the University of California at Berkeley, where Leary began his doctoral studies in the fall of 1947.

Leary arrived as both his field of study and the San Francisco Bay area were in the throngs of a postwar boom. Hundreds of thousands of GIs had passed through San Francisco on their way to serve in the Pacific, liked what they saw, and settled down in the Bay Area after the war. At the same time, thousands of those soldiers had returned from combat with serious psychological injuries, and the Veterans Administration faced a severe shortage of psychiatrists and clinical psychologists with the skills needed to treat them.

Meanwhile, more and more Americans had begun moving away from religious counseling and toward psychotherapy. Therapists were becoming the new high priests. In the spring of 1956, *Time* magazine put Sigmund Freud on its cover, signaling that the psychoanalytic movement had established mainstream credibility. By then, the practice of psychology was already undergoing changes that would transform the field in the 1960s and 1970s. As a graduate student, Leary was learning the trade as two leading agents of psychological change were coming onto the scene. Carl Rogers, one of the founders of the humanist psychology movement, was on the faculty at Ohio State. Rogers, along with such humanistic pioneers as Abraham Maslow, sought to move beyond behaviorism and traditional psychoanalysis and take a more humane, positive approach to psychology—helping individuals foster creativity and discover their "true selves." In Berkeley, Leary studied with Erik Erikson, the noted child psychologist, who believed that psychologically healthy individuals go through eight stages of life in which they learn to cultivate such qualities as hope, will, purpose, competence, fidelity, love, caring, and wisdom.

After getting his PhD from Berkeley in 1950, Leary helped start the Department of Psychology at Kaiser Hospital in nearby Oakland. The hospital began as a clinic for wartime shipyard workers employed by Henry Kaiser but would soon blossom into one of the nation's most innovative health-care providers. It was here that Leary began his lifelong friendship with Frank Barron, a Berkeley classmate and Kaiser colleague. Leary and Barron shared many interests. They both liked to drink and play tennis, and both were more interested in the writing of James Joyce than of Sigmund Freud. And they were both, as Tim liked to say, "half-crazed Irishmen."

Leary's career and life would veer so far off course in the 1960s and 1970s that it's easy to forget that he was once considered a rising star in mainstream psychology. He and Barron collaborated on a much-discussed 1955 study of 150 patients awaiting psychiatric treatment at Kaiser Hospital. They found that a third of those patients improved following traditional psychotherapy, a third deteriorated, and a third pretty much stayed the same. Those were the same results for a control group of patients who *did not receive any treatment.* It was not good news for the psychological establishment. Over the next five years, Leary would publish three works that—in retrospect—prefigure the controversial ideas and research methods he would develop in the aftermath of his psychedelic baptism in the summer of 1960.

He is best remembered in academic circles for his 1957 book, *The Interpersonal Diagnosis of Personality.* The book presents a statistical analysis of data collected from hundreds of patients in group therapy sessions. It lays out five levels of interpersonal communication and proposes a new way to look at personality types. Leary's work challenged the prevailing psychological theory of the time—behaviorism, which focused exclusively on observing, measuring, and modifying behavior. Leary argued that people have the power and freedom to change their unconscious reactions to external stimuli. To Leary, social interaction was a kind of game. People could be coached to become better players, and take power over their own lives. Tim devised a personality test that soon became known as "the Leary Circle," a self-aggrandizing title that sparked resentment among research psychologists who thought Leary had unfairly capitalized on their work.

Psychologist Herbert Kelman, who would later emerge as one of the fiercest critics of Leary and Alpert's drug research, came to teach at Harvard in 1957, two years before Leary was brought into the psychology department. Kelman had been impressed with Leary's early work, but he was not so enthralled by the man himself. At first, the two psychologists had a friendly relationship. Kelman and his wife helped Leary and his two kids find a place to live. But it didn't take long for Kelman to start seeing Leary as more of a showman than a scholar. Kelman spotted a troubling megalomania in Leary, who had grandiose ideas about redefining the entire practice of clinical psychology. He came to lecture at one of Kelman's classes and spent the whole time knocking traditional clinical psychology. Kelman found the lecture overly negative and destructive. He was not impressed with Leary's iconoclastic approach. Leary loved using the word *existential.* Kelman knew a thing or two about existential philosophy, and he decided that Leary clearly did not.

Leary may not have been an expert in existentialism, but he *was* having his own existential crisis. It started back in Berkeley, in 1955, with his wife's suicide. Three years later, in 1958, Leary escaped to

Europe with his two young children, sailing off to Spain aboard the SS *Independence* of the American Export Lines. He rented a villa on the Costa del Sol and sat down to write the great American novel. He didn't get far into the book. Leary got sick; deadly ill, with a mysterious disease that swelled up his face and caused giant blisters to erupt on his cheeks. Leary survived that ordeal, and in the spring of 1959 he relocated to Florence, setting up shop in a penthouse overlooking the red-tiled domes of the picturesque Tuscan city. It had a great view, but there was a problem. Leary was broke. He'd exhausted a small research grant and liquidated several insurance policies. He'd quit his Kaiser job. His own research back in Oakland had made him believe that traditional psychotherapy was a waste of time. That's when Frank Barron, his old drinking pal at Cal, showed up in Florence. Barron wouldn't shut up about some strange experiences he had after eating "magic mushrooms" down in Mexico. Frank went on and on about his revelations, about all the mystical insights and transcendental perspectives produced by the strange fungi. Leary actually started to worry that his old friend was losing his mind, or at least in danger of losing his academic credibility.

Frank Barron had some other news—some more-practical information that might help this destitute father of two find a job back in the States. Barron had run into one of their colleagues, Professor David McClelland of the Harvard Center for Personality Research, who just happened to be on sabbatical in Florence. McClelland had just read *The Interpersonal Diagnosis of Personality* and was very impressed with Leary's work. The next day, Leary found himself sitting down with McClelland over a bottle of Chianti. By the time they finished lunch, McClelland had offered him a job back at Harvard. As Leary remembers the conversation, McClelland told him, "There's no question that what you're advocating is the future of American psychology.

"You're spelling out front-line tactics," his new boss proclaimed. "You're just what we need to shake things up at Harvard."

Healer
Philadelphia
Summer 1942

Andrew Weil was born in Philadelphia on June 8, 1942. His parents were secular Jews and ran a hat shop and millinery supply house. As a young child, Andy liked to grow flowers in small pots and on a tiny plot of land behind their row house. It was a pastime he picked up from his mother and grandmother, and it would blossom into a lifelong interest in botany.

Andy was an only child. Both of his parents worked, so he spent a lot of time by himself. He had what child psychologists would call "a very active interior life." He'd make up stories in his mind, and the stories seemed as real as reality itself. The boundary between his imagination and the world around him was a thin one. As an adult, Andy would build a successful career around the idea that what one sees in one's mind can actually change physical reality—that the mind can heal the body. Weil would keep this conviction throughout his education, even through his years at Harvard Medical School.

Decades later, many of his old med-school colleagues would scoff at Weil's ideas about the human body healing itself through such far-out techniques as guided imagery, breathing exercises, and self-hypnosis. One of his old teachers from Harvard would eventually condemn him as a snake-oil salesman. But others in the American medical establishment would come to see that Weil was onto something—that mainstream Western medicine had seriously underestimated the connection between a patient's mental state and his physical health.

These were ideas that would resonate with many baby boomers, including those whose extraordinary experiences on psychedelic drugs forced them to reexamine conventional ideas about body, mind, and spirit. By the 1990s, Weil would preside over a natural-foods and alternative-heath-care empire that would include his own medical center, television series, vitamin business, cosmetics line, and a series of three health and diet books that would all reach the top of the *New York Times* best-seller list. By the dawn of the new millennium, Dr. Weil would be known by such monikers as "Mr. Natural" and "the CEO of alternative medicine in America."

Andy's first encounters with American medicine were positive ones. Growing up in the late 1940s and early 1950s, he had a family doctor who was just a three-block walk from his parents' home in northwest Philadelphia. He could tell that his general practitioner—who made house calls and rarely prescribed pharmaceutical drugs—loved his profession. He spent lots of time with his patients, and his example inspired Andy to start thinking about becoming a doctor when he grew up.

One of the boy's earliest childhood memories involves a hospital stay where he was given ether by an anesthesiologist. He remembers drifting off in a strange trance. Like many children, Andy experimented with various means of altering his state of consciousness—not through drugs, but by such practices as spinning around and around and whirling himself into a vertiginous stupor. In his first book, *The Natural Mind: A New Way of Looking at Drugs and Higher Consciousness,* Weil would cite these mindaltering games as evidence to support the book's major thesis: that the "desire to alter consciousness periodically is an innate, normal drive analogous to hunger or the sexual drive.

"Anyone who watches very young children without revealing his presence will find them regularly practicing techniques that induce striking changes in mental states," he would write. "To my knowledge these practices appear spontaneously among children of all societies, and I suspect that they have done so throughout history as well. In our society, children quickly learn to keep this sort of play out of sight of grownups, who instinctively try to stop them. The sight of a child being throttled into unconsciousness scares the parent, but the child seems to have a wonderful time."

Like most children coming of age in the 1950s, Weil learned that consuming alcoholic beverages was the socially accepted way to alter one's state of consciousness. He remembers his grandmother Mayme getting the giggles after downing an after-dinner Brandy Alexander. Little Andy loved those moments, and tried to intensify the effect by tickling his tipsy grandma. The giggles turned into uncontrollable laughter, which would go on for ten minutes or so, leaving the old lady flushed and wet with tears. His parents were often embarrassed by the outbursts, but not Andy. He got a terrific contact high from those games with grandma, and he always suspected that she was onto something. Growing up, he would be known as quite the practical jokester, a habit that allowed him plenty of opportunities to fall into that altered state of consciousness known as hysterical laughter. Decades later, he would still be advising patients to practice "laughter yoga."

No one in his family was a big drinker, but young Weil was allowed occasional sips of cocktails or after-dinner drinks. He didn't discover a real alcoholic high until his senior year in high school, when he started going to weekend drinking parties where the idea was to get as drunk as possible. But the novelty soon wore off. Weil still went to the parties, but he drank in order to fit in with the crowd, not to get smashed.

Andy was often lonely as a child, and he would remain something of a loner for his entire life. At the same time, his solitary childhood gave him a fiercely independent spirit. He learned how to operate on his own and think for himself. When he was a teenager attending Central High School in Philadelphia, one of his favorite stories was J. D. Salinger's "Teddy," the tale of a precocious, mystical boy who questions the advice given by conventional doctors, only to get noticed by scholars as a boy wonder. The short story unfolds on an ocean liner, where a professor is talking to the ten-year-old genius.

"Ever think you might like to do something in research when you grow up? Medical research, or something of that kind?"

Teddy answered, but without sitting down. "I thought about that once, a couple of years ago," he said. "I've talked to quite a few doctors." He shook his head. "That wouldn't interest me very much. Doctors stay too right on the surface."

Andy Weil turned into J. D. Salinger's Teddy.

At age seventeen, the year before he entered Harvard, Andy won a scholarship from the American Association for the United Nations and embarked on a nine-month trip around the world, living with families in Greece, Thailand, and India. One experience on that trip had a profound impact. It occurred in December 1959 in Calcutta about halfway through his year abroad. One night when the moon was full, Andy and a classmate wandered down to a small Hindu temple on the banks of the Hugli River. They were just starting to explore the shrine when Andy felt a hand on his right shoulder. He quickly turned and saw that an old sadhu, an Indian renunciate in rags and long beard, was reaching out to him. Before he could say a word, the temple caretaker let out the most extraordinary sound the boy had ever heard. *Ommmmm. Ommmmm. Ommmmm.* Andy looked with amazement into the old man's radiant face, shining there in the light of the moon. Later that evening, he and his friend would learn that they had just heard the sacred sound of *aum,* a healing tone that encompasses all the sounds of the universe. When he closed his eyes, the awestruck teenager could still feel the mysterious vibrations deep down in his soul.

Andy came home convinced that much of American culture and science was clueless about the rest of the world. There was another reality out there, one far more interesting than what they were talking about in high school. Over the summer before college, he came across an article in the *Philadelphia Evening Bulletin* about a southern California college student who had allegedly died from an overdose of mescaline. What got Weil's attention was not that the student had died, but that he'd been taking the drug to get inspiration for a class in creative writing. The article described how mescaline produces powerful visions—including "galaxies of exploding colors."

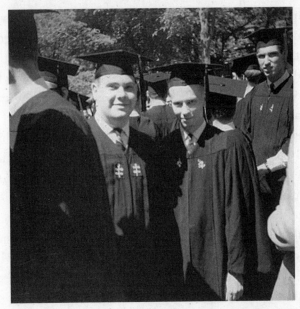

*Andrew Weil, (left) when he graduated from Harvard in 1964 (Photo courtesy of Andrew Weil.)*

That was something Andy Weil wanted to try. He couldn't find much at the local library about mescaline, but he did discover a six-year-old book by a British writer named Aldous Huxley. It was called *The Doors of Perception.* It describes Huxley's experience after ingesting a dose of mescaline in his home in the Hollywood hills in the spring of 1953. Huxley was sitting in his library, where his books began to take on a strange significance. "Red books, like rubies; emerald books; books bound in white jade; books of agate; of aquamarine, of yellow topaz; lapis lazuli books whose color was so intense, so intrinsically meaningful, that they seemed to be on the point of leaving the shelves to thrust themselves more insistently on my attention." Even the writer's gray flannel trousers came alive, supercharged with the "is-ness" of trousers. The draperies in his study became "so strange and dramatic that they catch the eye," inspiring a transformative appreciation of "the miraculous fact of sheer existence."

These descriptions of Huxley's visions still danced in Andy Weil's mind when he arrived at Harvard in the fall of 1960. At first, the young student had no idea what he wanted to study. (He'd wind up with a bachelor's degree in botany and an undergraduate thesis titled "The Use of Nutmeg as a Psychotropic Agent.") One of Weil's freshman classes was a sociology course taught by Professor David Riesman, for which Weil proposed a paper on American social attitudes toward psychoactive drugs.

Riesman was open to such topics. Ten years earlier, in 1950, he had published *The Lonely Crowd,* one of the most influential studies of the American character. Riesman had identified several American character types, including people who are mostly "other-directed" and those who are primarily "inner-directed." The 1950s, a decade that would become synonymous with unquestioning conformity, had seen the rise of the other-directed character—all those middle-class, upwardly mobile businessmen and consumers who focused on other people's opinions of them. By the early 1960s, however, more and more Americans were starting to follow an inner voice. There was a new kind of empathic individualism, a nonconformist mentality that would soon see full flowering in the psychedelic drug culture. One way to see this change is through film and theater—the social journey from *Death of a Salesman* to *Easy Rider.*

Weil discussed his idea for his class paper with one of Riesman's teaching assistants.

"If you're interested in studying psychoactive drugs, you're sure in the right place," the graduate student told him. "Go check out this psychologist who's working with David McClelland. His name's Leary, and he's into some pretty interesting stuff."

Weil couldn't believe his luck. He called and made an appointment to come over for his visit. Over the phone, Leary told Weil that he had a tiny office over at the Center for Research in Personality.

"We're easy to find," Leary said with a chuckle. "We're located at Five Divinity Avenue."

## Teacher
## Soochow, China
## Spring 1919

Huston Smith—a man who would devote his life to helping the materialist West understand the mysterious East—was born in Soochow (Suzhou), China, on May 31, 1919. His parents were Methodist missionaries, as were his mother's parents.

Huston's grandparents first set out in 1883 for the monthlong voyage from New York to China, settling down in Zhenjiang. Huston's father felt the missionary call while studying for his master's degree at Vanderbilt University, where he came across a group of young Christian activists, the Student Volunteer Movement, who had set out to "Christianize the world in this generation." One evening his father was listening to a recruiter who pulled a stopwatch from his vest pocket and proceeded to shock his audience with the bad news of how many Chinese souls were going to hell as each second passed. "Who among you are willing to join us to save those lost souls, to preach the Good News?" the orator asked, inspiring Huston's father to raise his hand.

His mother and father met at the Methodist university in Soochow, a city about fifty miles west of Shanghai. His father was teaching English at the university while learning Chinese. Their first son died at age two from one of the many infectious diseases that swept through the crowded city. Huston was the second of three other sons born in Soochow before his parents headed to the interior of the vast pagan nation, inspired to find a town "where Christ had never been preached."

They settled in Dzang Zok (Changshu), a small town about thirty miles north of Soochow. Huston's earliest memory as a very young child is of being on fire, a feeling that came from one of the raging fevers that would infect him and his brothers. Like Andrew Weil, whose earliest memories revolved around strange visions sparked by hospital anesthesia, Huston Smith recalls his childhood fevers as his first taste of an altered state of consciousness. His high fevers caused him to hallucinate and then feel like he was rising up out of his own body. His spirit rose up into the corner of the room, looking down at a sick little boy lying in bed. Then his body began to inflate like a giant balloon, filling the entire room.

Huston recovered, and learned to love the magic and misery of China. He'd often wake up in the middle of the night and walk outside to gaze up at the wonder of star-strewn skies. A few times, he woke up in the morning to find someone's unwanted infant left on the doorstep of his missionary parents' home.

Their house was the only one in town that had a porch. It smelled of roses from all the vines that covered the small veranda. A city wall encircled Dzang Zok, whose gates were locked after 10 P.M. to protect the town from warlords and their bandits. The narrow lanes in the crowded town were so compact that even as a boy Huston could stretch his arms far enough to touch the little row houses on either side of the street. As a boy, he was fascinated by the shamanism and superstition of Chinese popular religion. Empty bottles—nozzles pointed outward—lined the lintels of their small homes. They served as little canons mounted to warn demon spirits that they would be blown to pieces if they tried to enter the house and cause mischief.

When he was twelve years old, Huston was sent off to an American boarding school in Shanghai. He thought he was ready for the adventure, barely looking back as the little boat pulled away from the town dock and headed down the canal to the big city. He loved his first week, but on the weekends, when the pressure of classes was lifted, he'd sometimes walk out to the middle of the deserted athletic field, bury his face in his arms, and cry his heart out in homesickness. That devastating sadness lasted only a few weeks, but the memories of his childhood desperation would stay with him a lifetime.

Huston always assumed that he would follow his father into the Methodist ministry. His only role model in the little Chinese town was his father, so he grew up thinking that missionaries were what

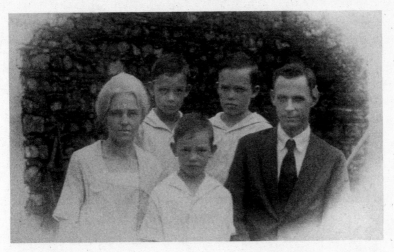

*Huston Smith stands behind his mother in a family photo taken in China in the 1920s. (Photo courtesy of Huston Smith.)*

missionary sons grew up to be. When he was seventeen years old, Smith set sail for his first visit to the United States. His destination was Central College in Fayette, Missouri, a small Bible college chosen by his father for Huston's missionary training. Smith had no idea what he was about to experience. He couldn't believe his eyes. It was just a little Missouri town of three thousand people, but to Huston it was bright lights, big city.

Smith had planned to return to rural China as a missionary—plans that lasted about two weeks once he landed in the United States. The obvious alternative was to stay and find his calling as a Methodist minister, but after two years on that track, Smith decided that teaching—not preaching—was his true calling. Like his father, Huston would be ordained as a minister in the United Methodist Church. But the son would reject the theology of the father. Huston Smith had no desire to "Christianize the world."

Huston's theological ideas had begun to shift at Central College, where he met a philosophy professor who introduced the young Bible student to the work of Henry Nelson Wieman, an influential liberal theologian at the University of Chicago Divinity School. Smith was very much taken by Wieman's ideas, but he was even more infatuated with the professor's daughter, Kendra. They met in the summer of 1941 at a packed campaign rally for Norman Thomas, a Presbyterian minister who was running for president on the Socialist Party of America ticket. Huston had gone to college with Kendra's brother. At first, she was not too sure about her new suitor. Kendra was a sophisticated young lady. She was already calling herself a Buddhist. "Huston's parents are *very* conservative," she told a friend. "They are set against cards and dancing. His mother dresses up to the neck. Huston doesn't know a thing about sex."

Huston and Kendra were married in 1943. Kendra was just twenty years old, and pregnant within three weeks of taking her vows. Their marriage would produce three daughters and span seven decades.

Huston was more faithful to his wife than he was to his father-in-law's philosophy. Wieman (1884–1975) was originally ordained into the Presbyterian Church but later found more sympathetic fellowship among the Unitarians. He was strongly influenced by the ideas of the mathematician-philosopher Alfred North Whitehead and the educational reformer John Dewey. He developed a theology known as "naturalistic theism," which sought to reconcile religion with the scientific worldview. Huston was still working on his doctoral thesis when he began to question the philosophy of the Harvard-educated Wieman, who argued that the only world we can describe with any certainty is the world of nature—the objective reality we experience through our senses or through the rigors of scientific investigation. Wieman's intellectual world left little room for investigations into the supernatural and the metaphysical.

Smith lost his faith in Wieman's ideas following a chance encounter with a man he would later describe as "the best-kept secret of the twentieth century." Huston was studying at the University of California at Berkeley, writing a section of his dissertation that dealt with the problem of pain. He'd gone to the library looking for books with the word *pain* in the title, and one title leapt out from the card catalog. It was *Pain, Sex and Time,* a strange and somewhat convoluted book written by a man named Gerald Heard.

Heard (1889–1971) was a prolific British writer and radio com-mentator who came to the United States with Aldous Huxley in 1937. Heard had been offered the chair of historical anthropology at Duke University, but he soon abandoned that post and settled in the Santa Ana Mountains of southern California to found Trabuco College, a short-lived institute focusing on the study of comparative religion. Heard was among a group of California literati to discover an Indian guru named Swami Prabhavananda, who came to the United States in 1923 and founded the Vedanta Society of South-ern California in 1930. Heard became a serious student of yoga and meditation—spiritual practices he believed would result in an evolution of higher consciousness in the human race. He would later donate all of the Trabuco College buildings and real estate to the Vedanta Society.

Huston Smith became a Gerald Heard junkie. He devoured *Pain, Sex and Time,* which was published in 1939, and dedicated himself to reading every word Heard had ever written—no small task considering that the British philosopher had written more than two dozen books. What Smith found so exhilarating about Heard's work was his thesis that evolution was not over—that hu-manity was on the cusp of a breakthrough in consciousness. Reli-gious mystics were a kind of spiritual scouting party, showing the way forward.

It wasn't until the end of World War II that Smith was able to fulfill his vow to meet the man whose ideas had changed his life. Huston had just finished school and had begun his first teach-ing job in Denver. He had finished phase one of his Gerald Heard initiation by reading all of the man's published works. Unaware that Heard had just started his own college in southern Califor-nia, Smith wrote to the British writer in care of his publisher. But Heard soon answered and said he'd be glad to meet with Huston at his monastery southeast of Los Angeles. Smith, still paying off his debts from graduate school, was so broke that he didn't own a car, but that didn't stop him from hitchhiking all the way from Denver to Heard's hideaway in the Santa Ana Mountains. Heard welcomed Smith upon his arrival and invited him to share a meal. After supper they went out and sat together on a large rock on the side of the canyon. They just sat there in silence, gazing at the barren canyon walls. Huston suddenly realized there was nothing he needed to ask the man. It was enough to just sit together with him on the edge of the canyon.

That evening was the beginning of a long and fruitful association between Huston Smith and Gerald Heard, and through Heard, between Huston and Aldous Huxley, who would play a key role in the events about to unfold at Harvard. Toward the end of their 1948 meeting at Trabuco Canyon, Smith asked Heard if he knew how he could get in touch with Aldous Huxley. Heard thought it was a splendid idea. After all, this young man had hitch-hiked all the way from Denver to see him. "Let me give you his phone number in Los Angeles," Heard said. "Aldous always likes meeting people who share our interests."

Huston headed into Los Angeles, and when he got there he pulled out the little scrap of paper Heard had given him with Huxley's number. Huston phoned the number, and a house sitter answered. She explained that Huxley and his wife, Maria, had escaped to their little hideaway in the Mojave Desert, but she was sure that the couple would not mind a call from a friend of Gerald Heard's. Huston scribbled the second number down on the scrap of paper and dialed the number. Huxley answered the phone.

"Gerald Heard thought we should meet? Then we should most certainly meet," Huxley said. "Let me give you directions."

"What? You have no car? Well, here's what you do. Take the bus straight out toward San Bernardino. We're about half way across the desert to the left of the highway. You'll see a cabin. It's the only thing out there. Tell the driver you're looking for the ruins of Llano."

Huxley and his wife had moved out to the desert during the war and were living among the ruins of Llano del Rio, a failed socialist utopian colony. Aldous had grown tired of the celebrity scene in Hollywood, where he'd been writing screenplays, and had come to the desert to write *The Perennial Philosophy,* an anthology and commentary on the insights of the great mystical traditions. Huxley's ideas would be among those to inspire Smith to write *The Religions of Man,* which was first published in 1958 and would sell more than two and a half million copies before a fiftieth anniversary edition of the work, now called *The World's Religions,* was issued in 2009.

But here Huston was, six decades earlier, in the summer of 1948, on a bus rumbling into the Mojave Desert. Suddenly, he saw the place! There it was, more of a shack than a house. It stood under a clump of poplar trees planted alongside an irrigation ditch. It was a little oasis of vines and fruit trees, and there was the tall, lanky frame of Aldous Huxley, standing outside, waving at the bus to San Bernardino. Huxley welcomed Smith into the cabin and introduced him to Maria, who was cleaning up the place and getting ready for the arrival of their mysterious visitor. Huston remembers helping the beautiful Maria make up their bed and sweep out some sand that had blown in through the open door. Smith, a young man still in his twenties, couldn't believe he was actually standing there in the hideaway of Aldous and Maria Huxley.

Aldous and Huston went for a walk in the desert. Huxley talked about the symbolic power of the boundless sand—how, like snow, it spread its sameness over the multiplicity of the world. He spoke of the prophets of the Old Testament, the Desert Fathers, and how they can still speak to us today. It was a brief visit, just like the previous day's pilgrimage to see Gerald Heard, but the two encounters would shape the life of Huston Smith. Before saying good-bye to Aldous and Maria, Huston mentioned that he had just landed a new job teaching at Washington University in St. Louis.

"Well," Huxley replied, "if you're moving to St. Louis, I know of a very good swami there that you should meet."

Smith wasn't sure what a swami was, but he pulled out his little scrap of paper and wrote down the name, which sounded more like a sentence than a name. Swami Satprakashananda. Aldous spelled

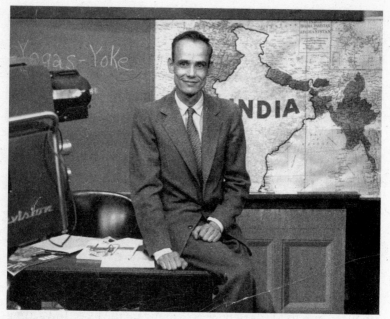

*Huston Smith on TV, 1958.*

it out for him. S-A-T-P-R-A-K-A-S-H-A-N-A-N-A-D-A. Shortly after his arrival, Smith would look up the St. Louis swami and visit his ashram. Within a few years, the popular religion professor at Washington University would find himself serving as both the president of the local Vedanta Society *and* associate minister at a local Methodist congregation. His life path was set—teaching, preaching, and exploring his own spiritual path.

Smith soon developed his own method for talking about other people's religious beliefs and spiritual practices. He would seek to understand them from the inside out. His search for the essence of a religious faith would take him past the outer forms and rituals and into the mystical core of Buddhism, Taoism, Hinduism, and other major world religions. This was back in the 1950s, when most Americans had never heard of the Dalai Lama or the Five Pillars of Islam. That was about to change. In 1955, Smith would host a series of programs on world religions for the National Educational Television network, the precursor to PBS. Viewers across America gathered around small, flickering black-and-white screens to hear the rail-thin religion professor from St. Louis explain the mysteries of the Bhagavad Gita. Looking back at tapes of the old programs, there's something very quaint, almost comical, about Smith's presentation. It was the early days of television. Smith stood alongside a desk and chalkboard, writing down mysterious words like *yoga*. Then he removed his shoes, flashed a sheepish grin, and climbed up onto the wooden desk to assume the lotus position. Two years later, Smith would make his first pilgrimage to India, where he would become entranced with the teeming wonder of it all. He couldn't quite explain the feeling, he told friends, but "part of me seems to have been here from the beginning."

In 1958, Smith's rising popularity as an authority on the religions of the world landed him a job as professor of Asian philosophy at the prestigious Massachusetts Institute of Technology, just down the road from Harvard. Ten years had passed since their meeting in the Mojave, but Smith was one of the several MIT faculty members who would invite Aldous Huxley to come to Cambridge in the fall of 1960 to help the institute celebrate its one hundredth anniversary.

Huxley was paid nine thousand dollars to give seven public lectures as the Centennial Carnegie Visiting Professor in Humanities. They were held in the Kresge Oval, a stunning example of midcentury modern architecture whose elegant, sweeping roof—a thin-shelled, copper-clad structure—covers a wall of windows and rises gracefully from the campus green. It was still a new building on the evening of October 5, 1960, when Aldous Huxley walked onstage for his first lecture. All 1,238 seats were filled. When the fire marshal tried to clear the aisles of student standees from Harvard and MIT, Huxley not only asked that they be allowed to stay, but invited two hundred of them to share the stage with him. Huxley's lectures were so popular that extra police were brought in to handle the traffic jams. He and Huston would spend a lot of time together during those two months in Cambridge, with Huston accompanying Huxley on many of his out-of-town engagements.

In the interval between their encounter in the Mojave and their reunion at MIT, Huxley had experimented with mescaline and written *The Doors of Perception,* the first comprehensive account of the psychedelic experience by a popular English writer. Smith had been studying and writing about religious mysticism for more than a decade, but he never actually had a full-blown mystical experience. During one of their errands outside Cambridge, Huston asked Huxley if he had any idea how he could find someone who would give him those mysterious drugs he'd written about in *The Doors of Perception.*

"Oh, Huston, thanks for reminding me," Huxley replied. "There's this interesting chap over at Harvard I've been meaning to tell you about. I think you'd like to meet him. His name is Leary. Tim Leary. Remind me to give you his phone number."

# CHAPTER TWO

# Turn On

Trickster
Cuernavaca, Mexico
Summer 1960

Timothy Leary brought the bowl of mushrooms up to his nose and sniffed. The smell reminded him of musty New England basements, or perhaps a downed tree rotting in a damp forest. It was now or never. He slowly placed one of the black moldy things in his mouth and followed up fast with a cold chaser of Mexican beer. The mushrooms tasted worse than they smelled—bitter and stringy. Before he had time to change his mind, he stuffed the rest of them into his mouth, washing the mess down with that more familiar, and refreshing, alcoholic intoxicant.

It was supposed to just be a regular summer vacation, some time to relax before starting the new academic year. Leary and his son, Jack, now ten years old, scouted out the city of Cuernavaca and found a villa for rent—a rambling white stucco house with scarlet trim, next to a golf course on the road to Acapulco. Cuernavaca, whose name comes from an Aztec word for "place near trees," has been known in more recent times as the "city of eternal spring." Its temperate year-round climate made the place a popular getaway spot for many famous Americans, including Hollywood heiress Barbara Hutton, Chicago crime boss Sam Giancana, and the German-born humanistic psychologist Eric Fromm, who studied Mexican social customs in a village just down the road from the Leary villa. Professor David McClelland, the man who offered Leary his new post at Harvard, was on retreat and working on a book in nearby Tepozlan, about ten miles away. But the scholar who would have the most impact on Leary's summer vacation—and the rest of his life—was a University of Mexico linguist and anthropologist named Lothar Knauth, who was in the area translating ancient Aztec texts written in Nahuatl.

Leary was renting the Spanish-style villa—named "Casa del Moros" after a wealthy Arab who built the place—with two friends from San Francisco, semanticist Dick Dettering and his pregnant wife, Ruth. They had settled in and were awaiting the arrival of Frank Barron and Richard Alpert. Knauth had been hanging around the villa, enjoying the swimming pool and the lively company. In one of his conversations with Leary, Knauth mentioned that he knew a woman named Crazy Juana, an old *curandera,* a Mexican shaman, who collected magic mushrooms off the slopes of Toluca, a nearby volcano. Leary remembered how Barron had been talking last year in Italy about the wonders of these mysterious fungi. Maybe that was just the ingredient they needed to spice up their summer vacation at Casa del Moros.

"Why don't you see if you can find some," he told Knauth.

Leary's mushroom connection delivered on the afternoon of August 9, 1960.

Botanists classify these fungi as *Psilocybe cubensis,* but the Aztecs called them *teonanacatl,* the flesh of the gods. Psilocybin mushrooms, and the secretive indigenous religion that surrounds them, had been mostly unknown to the American public until an event three years earlier, when *Life* magazine published a long and sympathetic story in its issue of June 10, 1957. The piece was written by R. Gordon Wasson, a New York banker and amateur mycologist who liked to travel the world with his Russian-born wife and search for exotic fungi. The richly illustrated article recounts the adventures that Wasson and his photographer friend Allan Richardson had in southern Mexico in the summer of 1955 when they became "the first white men in recorded history to eat the divine mushrooms."

With the help of a local guide, Wasson and Richardson found a bountiful harvest in a damp ravine in the Mixeteco Mountains. They brought some of the musty plants to the thatched-roofed adobe home of Eva Mendez, a local *curandera*. "We showed our mushrooms to the woman and her daughter," Wasson writes. "They cried out in rapture over the firmness, the fresh beauty and abundance of our young specimens."

Sitting beside an altar adorned with flowers and icons depicting Jesus and his baptism in the River Jordan, Wasson ate twelve mushrooms and began a nightlong journey into worlds he thought he never knew, scenes that "seemed more real to me than anything I had ever seen with my own eyes.

"They were in vivid color, always harmonious. They began with art motifs, angular such as might decorate carpets or textiles or wallpaper of the drawing board of an architect. Then they evolved into palaces with courts, arcades, gardens—resplendent palaces all laid over with semiprecious stones. Then I saw a mythological beast drawing a regal chariot. Later it was as though the walls of our house had dissolved, and my spirit had flown forth, and I was suspended in mid-air viewing landscapes of mountains, with camel caravans advancing slowly across the slopes, the mountains rising tier above tier to the very heavens."

Five years later, sitting by the pool of his rented Mexican villa, Leary had his own encounter with the flesh of the gods. Dick Dettering and a couple of other guests joined him for the mushroom trip, while two people at the pool party decided to abstain. One was the pregnant Ruth Dettering, who was concerned about the effects the drug would have on her unborn child. The other abstainer was a friend of a friend who had shown up at the villa the previous night. Leary called him Whiskers. He suffered from nervous fits, and decided that an encounter with psilocybin mushrooms might drive him over the psychotic edge.

Leary started coming onto the drug. At first, he couldn't stop laughing. There was Whiskers, sitting by the pool in bathing trunks pulled over flowered undershorts. To top it off, he was wearing green garters, black socks, and leather shoes. Whiskers had decided to take notes while the rest of the crew tripped off to Mushroom Land. So there was Whiskers, bent over a notepad, scribbling away like some Viennese shrink on speed. Leary could not stop laughing. *Oh, the pomposity of scholars,* he thought, *the impudence of the mind.* Tim got up and staggered into the house, then back out to the pool on rubbery legs. Suddenly, he remembered the kids. *Who was watching the kids? What would the kids think?* He called over to the sober Ruth. "This is hitting us hard," Leary told her. "You may have six psychotic nuts on your hands. I think you should send the kids downtown to the movies, and the maid, too. Get her out of here. And lock the gates. Stay close, and for God's sake, keep an eye on us."

Leary was losing it. Someone asked, "How do you feel?" Tim couldn't speak. It was all too much. Everything around him started taking on the shimmer and glimmer of jeweled patterns. *How* do *I feel? Far away. Gone. Far. Far. Gone. Drifting off into a cavern of sea light.* Making his way back to the house, he fell on the bed, into the arms of another woman who had taken the mushrooms. *Bodies like warm foam rubber. Marshmallow flesh. Mermaids. Laughing. Poking fingers through bikini lace. Quicksand flesh. Dark hair. Ponytail. Cherokee princess. Hummingbird words buzz from mouth. Stop talking. Look outside. God! The undulating sea! Deep. Plants twirling together. Not even the plants know which leaf, which stem, belongs to which. Interconnected. Giant jungle palm time. Whoa! Oh!! My God!!!*

Everything was quivering with life, even inanimate objects. Leary saw Nile palaces, Hindu temples, Babylonian boudoirs, Bedouin pleasure tents. Then came silk gowns breathing color and mosaics of flaming emeralds, followed by jeweled Moorish serpents.

Three hours passed in an instant.

At one point, Leary realized that some other friends had shown up from Acapulco. He slid back into the old reality, not wanting to return, but knowing he had to play host and that he was almost sober enough to pull it off. "We took some mushrooms," he explained to his startled guests. "Absolutely amazing! Why don't you guys go into the kitchen and make yourselves a drink. We'll get some supper in a bit."

Another hour passed, and Leary was back from his visionary voyage. Seven psilocybin mushrooms and an ice-cold bottle of Carta Blanca. That's all it took. Leary was forced to confront the fragile nature of his beliefs. The mushroom ride shattered the foundation of his philosophy of life and his view of himself. What we call "reality" was just a social fabrication. He would later call his trip "the deepest religious experience of my life."

Timothy Leary returned from Mexico and immediately set up the Harvard Psilocybin Project. The idea was to recruit graduate students and faculty members from the many colleges, seminaries, and universities in the Boston area. They would take a controlled dose of psilocybin, the active ingredient in the magic mushroom, and then write up reports about their experiences. Leary was thoroughly convinced that psychedelic drugs would revolutionize the practice of psychology.

His project was officially part of the university, but its most important activities occurred within the walls of Leary's rented home at 64 Homer Street, just across the Charles River from Harvard, in the leafy Boston suburb of Newton. The spacious, three-story home sits atop a hill overlooking a neighborhood park and baseball diamond. A wealthy French bicycle manufacturer built it in 1893. Three large fireplaces radiate from its central chimney, warming wood-paneled rooms on the ground floor. The fireplaces were all ablaze during the psychedelic drug experiments Leary conducted over the long winter nights of late 1960 and early 1961. Today, you can still find burn marks that the absentminded professor left in the hardwood floor—physical evidence of the fire that burned in Leary's soul for the psychedelic revolution he was about to declare.

By the summer of 1960, Leary had completed the first year of his three-year Harvard contract. He was just getting used to the idea that he was now a single father. Some semblance of normalcy was returning to his life, but the mushroom visions were still dancing in his head when Leary returned to Harvard and the Center for Personality Research. Suddenly, he was more interested in metaphysics than clinical psychology.

Leary knew about Harvard's extraordinary history as a center for mainline psychological inquiry. After all, the father of American psychology, the great William James, spent his entire academic career at Harvard, teaching physiology, anatomy, psychology, and philosophy between the years 1873 and 1907. William was the son of Henry James Sr., the American theologian whose Cambridge home stood in the heart of the old Harvard College campus—where the Harvard Faculty Club stands today.

But there's another psychological tradition here, and it's a legacy Leary would later claim as his own—a tradition of "wondrous internal paganism," a rebel history of transcendentalism, mysticism, and self-reliance.

Every day on his way to work, Leary would walk by the Cambridge Swedenborg Chapel, a stately Gothic-revival sanctuary built by the founder of the university's school of architecture. It stands, in part, as a monument to Henry James Sr., who is best remembered for rejecting his father's stern Presbyterianism and finding a spiritual home in Swedenborgianism, a religious tradition founded by Emanuel Swedenborg, an eighteenth-century Swedish mystic and scientist. The other major influence in the life of the elder James would come through his association with former members of Brook Farm, who ran a utopian socialist commune in nearby Roxbury, Massachusetts, between 1841 and 1847. Those same years saw the births of two of Henry's sons, the famous ones: William, the psychologist-philosopher; and Henry James Jr., the American writer known for his 1881 novel *The Portrait of a Lady* and other works.

William James laid the foundation for American psychology in 1890 with the publication of his classic text, *The Principles of Psychology*. But the book that would establish the mystical tradition later claimed by Leary and Alpert—James's philosophical masterpiece, *The Varieties of Religious Experience*—appeared twelve years later, in 1902. Those writings reveal that Leary and Alpert were not the first Harvard psychologists to be transformed by mind-altering drugs. *The Varieties of Religious Experience* praises the mystical qualities produced by two drugs popular in that era—alcohol and nitrous oxide. "Sobriety diminishes, discriminates, and says no; drunkenness expands, unites and says yes. It is, in fact, the great exciter of the *Yes* function in man," James wrote of the alcoholic high. "To the poor and the unlettered it stands in the place of symphony concerts and of literature. . . . The drunken consciousness is one bit of the mystic consciousness, and our total opinion of it must find its place in our opinion of that larger whole."

Leary, a heavy drinker who blamed alcoholism for three generations of misery in his Irish clan, was more taken by the book's ode to nitrous oxide, which James used to "stimulate the mystical consciousness in an extraordinary degree.

"Depth beyond depth of truth seems revealed to the inhaler," James wrote. "I know of more than one person who is persuaded that in the nitrous oxide trance we have a genuine metaphysical transformation. . . . Our normal waking consciousness, rational consciousness as we call it, is but one special type of consciousness, whilst all about it, parted from it by the filmiest of screens, there lie potential forms of consciousness entirely different."

In a rare show of modesty, Leary would later say that his own descriptions of the wonders of LSD intoxication pale when compared with the revelations of William James. The father of American psychology, Leary quipped, "corrupted many a mind by describing the glories of nitrous oxide in far more colorful prose than the most intoxicated Irishman."

Leary came back to Harvard as a man transformed. There was no way he was going back to his old life, to his old ways of doing things. His new boss, David McClelland, was just finishing up his book *The Achieving Society,* a psychological investigation into why some societies prosper and others fall apart. Surely David McClelland would understand the importance of these insights. He would certainly agree that these psychedelic experiences could be used to further the goal they both shared—to humanize the profession of psychology and foster an enlightened, compassionate society.

He didn't.

Leary saw unlimited possibilities.

McClelland saw administrative hurdles and political problems.

Leary suddenly realized that there was no way to convey the power of the mushroom vision. It was something you had to experience firsthand. It was something every man would have to try for himself.

### Teacher
### Newton, Massachusetts
### New Year's Day, 1961

For Huston Smith, there were many things to celebrate at the close of the year, many blessings for which to give thanks. Aldous Huxley had just finished his series of lectures at the Massachusetts Institute of Technology, the latest and most prestigious university to include Smith on its faculty. America had just elected a young and vibrant Democrat—a Massachusetts senator *and* a Harvard man—to begin the decade as the new president of the United States. Smith's new book, *The Religions of Man,* was starting to sell and find its niche as an introductory textbook in religious-studies courses at colleges around the country.

But there was something missing from Huston's life. He'd been teaching and writing about the mystical experience—the root of all

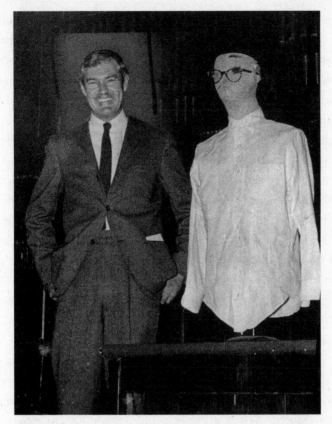

*Timothy Leary still had the buttoned-down look in this photo taken at a Boston club in early 1966. (Photo by John Landers, Boston Globe.)*

religion—for more than a decade. He had his yoga and meditation practice, the spiritual regime suggested by the good swamis of the Vedanta Society. There had been little flashes of insight, tempting tastes of the state of consciousness achieved by great masters of mysticism, but Smith had never had the full-blown mystical experience Huxley described in *The Doors of Perception.*

Huxley first crossed paths with Leary during his fall sojourn in Cambridge. At first, the novelist-turned-mystic had great hopes for the psychedelic research Leary had just begun. They met over dinner at a Boston restaurant on Election Day—the very night

John F. Kennedy was elected president of the United States. Joining Leary and Huxley at the table was Humphrey Osmond, a British scientist who had already done extensive psychedelic drug research. Osmond had run into Leary at a conference in Boston and had offered to arrange the meeting with the famous British writer. Leary jumped at the chance. He arrived at the restaurant wearing a gray flannel suit. He knew that his dinner partners were the real experts in psychedelic drugs. After all, Osmond was the man who had first introduced Huxley to mescaline, the trip that inspired Aldous to write *The Doors of Perception*. All through dinner, Leary tried as hard as he could not to come across as too much of an eager beaver. He may have overdone it. After Tim left the restaurant, Huxley and Osmond started talking about whether Leary was the right man to carry the psychedelic torch.

"Seems like a solid chap," Huxley said. "What do you think?"

"I don't know," Osmond replied. "Seems a bit stuffy, don't you think?"

"Yes," Aldous said. "Perhaps."

It wouldn't take long for the two Brits to see that their first impression was an extraordinarily inaccurate assessment of Timothy Leary. Stuffy? When it came to his attitude toward psychedelic drugs, *messianic* was closer to the mark. A couple of years later, Huxley and Osmond would have another conversation about the man who was fast becoming the world's most infamous spokesman for the psychedelic cause. "I'm very fond of Timothy," Huxley would say, "but why, oh why, does he have to be such an ass!"

Huxley and Osmond would part ways with Leary over disagreements as to the best way to change the world through psychedelic drugs. Leary wanted to turn on the whole world. Huxley was more cautious. He thought elite opinion makers and trendsetters should have the experience, which might be too much of a revelation for the common man.

Huston Smith would eventually fall into the Huxley camp, but in the fall of 1960, the enthusiastic religion scholar was ready to join the Leary crusade. After all, none other than Aldous Huxley had recommended Timothy Leary as the perfect person to guide Huston Smith into these mysterious realms of higher consciousness. Smith made the phone call, and the two men arranged to meet for lunch at the Harvard Faculty Club.

On the appointed day, Huston walked into the dining room. Leary greeted him with a warm handshake and a wide grin. *What a charmer,* Huston thought. Leary was wearing fine English tweeds atop gleaming white tennis shoes. *Now there's a man with flair.*

It didn't take long for Leary and Smith to start talking about the drug research.

"Well, you know, Tim," Huston said, "I've never tried these substances."

"Then you are perfectly qualified," Leary replied. "All you have to do is to write up a two- or three-page account about your experience the day after our session. We're really looking for someone who knows something about mysticism to look over all these reports we've collected. I'm a psychologist, not a religion scholar. I was hoping to get Aldous to do it, but he didn't have time. He said, 'Talk to Huston. He knows all about that.'"

Smith was more than happy to help out.

"I don't know what *you* are doing," he told Leary. "I *do* know about the mystical experience, but not about it being engendered this way. So I guess I'd better find out before I start pontificating about it."

"I can certainly arrange that," Leary replied.

So the two professors pulled out their date books and tried to find a completely open day they could devote to the experience. Leary had already learned how important it was for his research subjects to have at least a full day and night set aside with no distractions to fully appreciate and absorb the effects of the drug. Leary and Smith both had busy schedules in October and November. Then the holidays were coming up.

Finally, with a twinkle in his eye, Leary said, "How about New Year's Day?"

They had a date.

Smith thought it might be a good idea for his wife, Kendra, to come along for the ride. "The more the merrier," Leary said. On the appointed day, they arrived at the Leary home in Newton. They got there just after noon. Joining them were Frank Barron, the codirector of the Harvard Psilocybin Project, and Dr. George Alexander, a psychiatrist who was present to handle any psychological emergencies that might arise. After a little small talk, Leary pulled out some capsules and explained that one was a mild dose, two were average, and three were recommended for those who wanted a fuller experience of what the drug could offer. Kendra took three. Huston was more cautious at first, taking one capsule, but then downing another in half an hour, when nothing seemed to be happening.

After about an hour, Smith started feeling some tension in his legs, which then started to twitch. He decided that he had better lie down on the couch in Leary's large, comfortable living room. Aware that he would have to write a report on his experience, Huston tried desperately to pay attention to the exact moment when he passed into the visionary stage. That would prove to be impossible. His whole sense of time started to shift. Something was radically different about his thoughts and feelings. Everything that popped into his mind seemed strange, weird, uncanny, significant, and terrifying beyond belief. The drug was like a psychological prism. Suddenly he could see the infinitely complex and layered psychological ingredients that make up normal consciousness. These sensation-impressions were refracted, spread out as if by a spectroscope, into layers. How would he be able to describe these layers upon layers, these worlds within worlds? This was all beyond words. There was no way he could look back in the morning and describe all this. That would be impossible once he lost this new power of perception.

Huston's trip was awe inspiring, but it was not pleasurable. Everything in his mind seemed to be infinitely significant, but also strangely terrifying. At one point, he remembered that he had a body. Or did he? It felt like his body was laid out, half dead, on a slab, cool and slightly moist. But what was the connection between his body, mind, and spirit? His body would function only if his spirit chose to return to it, infuse it, and animate it. What if it didn't return? And why should it?

Leary walked into his living room to check on his subject. He could tell Huston was not having a good time. He had lain here for hours in a comatose terror. At one point, he cried out to Leary.

"Tim," Huston yelled. "I hope you know what you are playing around with because if I mount one step higher the terror is just going to explode my body and you'll be left with a corpse on your divan."

Leary walked over to the couch to reassure him that everything was OK.

"You'll be fine, Huston," Leary said. "I can guarantee you that I won't find a corpse on my couch."

"I know," Smith replied. "I have a family and I do not want to leave this life at this point. But I know with every conviction that I could if I wanted and you would have a corpse here on your divan."

Huston went back into a kind of trance, lying on the couch in silent, dazed contemplation. Leary offered tea. Huston didn't drink it. Fruit. It went uneaten. Words of encouragement and support. Huston failed to respond. Leary was afraid that he'd blown it. He knew Aldous Huxley and Huston Smith would be key allies in his psychedelic revolution, and now he'd sent the influential religion professor off on a bad trip.

Huston knew from reading Huxley that these were "heaven and hell" drugs. They can produce joy and terror—often in the same trip. That realization helped settle him down. At one point, he sat up on the couch and began to gaze into a blazing fire Leary had built to warm the room. Huston could hear soft voices in the next room, where Tim was talking to Barron. Huston was coming back to the old world. He'd made it back. His mind was reconnecting with his body.

Later that night, after Huston and Kendra had left, Leary was depressed. He was convinced that the night had been a failure, and blamed himself for his lack of experience in running these visionary sessions. He had lost his one chance to get the noted religion expert on board.

Leary was wrong. Kendra knew that Huston was mostly just kidding when he started talking about turning into a corpse on the sofa. Kendra did have to drive her husband home as he still seemed a bit stoned. "Such a sense of awe," he said in the car. "It was exactly what I was looking for."

Kendra was equally blown away by the experience. "I had this whole other sense of time," she said. "It was like I suddenly sensed eons and eons of time. It was like you're cleansing the doors of perception."

Huston's first trip inspired him to join the Leary team and take a leadership role in the research project for the next three years. It was more than a team, really. It felt like family. Sharing psychedelic drugs can forge a strong bond. Psychedelic partners often share a vision of another reality, and are never quite the same again. They join the club. Smith began to feel more connected to the twenty or so professors and graduate students on the psilocybin project than to anyone else in the academic community or in his church. They felt like the early explorers of Africa. They were discovering a whole new world that was spiritual, ephemeral, but at the same time felt more solid, more real, than everyday reality.

Over time, Smith, like Huxley, would come to question the zeal Leary and Alpert employed to spread the psychedelic gospel. Smith and another theologian on the team, Walter Houston Clark, joined forces with Leary and Alpert to form the International Federation for Internal Freedom, known to those in the know as "if . . . if." But Clark and Smith would eventually part ways with the two men who would become forever associated with the great adventure at Harvard.

Leary and Alpert were antiestablishment rebels. Walter and Huston thought of themselves as reformers, not revolutionaries. They were not ready to give up on the university.

———————

Huston Smith had come to MIT in 1958. He was thirty-nine years old and just hitting his stride as a scholar and commentator on the world's religions. Nearly five decades later, he sits in a sunny window in the living room of his home in Berkeley, California. He's still married to Kendra, but he's an old man now. He has trouble hearing, and with the help of a walker he can barely make it from his study to his living-room chair. But when he tells the story of that New Year's Day in Timothy Leary's living room, his eyes widen and he seems to lose ten years.

"What a way to start the sixties," he says, laughing.

## Seeker
### Newton, Massachusetts
### February 1961

Richard Alpert would have taken the magic mushrooms in Mexico with the rest of the gang, back in the summer of 1960, but he arrived a few days *after* Leary's first trip. Everyone was still aglow in the aftermath of the experience, but the mushrooms were gone. Richard would have to wait nearly nine months before he got his own psychedelic baptism back home in Timothy Leary's living room.

Back in Mexico in the summer of 1960, Leary was still feeling the mystic wonder of it all when he met Alpert at the Mexico City airport. Richard had quite an adventure just getting there. He'd just bought his flying teacher's Cessna and had decided to fly from San Francisco to Mexico City—over the startled objections of his instructor.

"There's no way you can do that," his teacher warned. "That's a really difficult airport to fly into. Traffic control is a mess down there."

"Don't worry," Alpert said. "I'll be fine."

He bought the plane on a Saturday and flew down on Sunday. He had not told his flight teacher he was going to fly down *tomorrow*. If he had he probably wouldn't have gotten the keys. Alpert had already rounded up a Stanford anthropologist who needed a lift to Mexico, but he didn't tell him he had just bought the Cessna the day before. Mexico City is at a high elevation, making it a difficult place to land. His passenger sat next to Alpert with a terrified look on his face as Richard dodged other airplanes on his approach.

"Don't worry," Alpert said. "We'll be fine."

They arrived and found Leary waiting in the terminal. Richard was eager to tell Tim about the terrors of his airplane trip, but it turned out Leary had an even more amazing trip to talk about.

They stood in the lobby as Alpert told the story about buying the plane and flying down to Mexico the next day.

"That's quite a trip, Richard," Leary said. "You know, I've been doing some flying myself—internally."

They got to the villa, and all the guests were sitting around the pool talking up the mushrooms. But the magic fungi were gone, and no one knew how to find Crazy Juana and score some more. Meanwhile, Leary was already planning his mushroom research project and wanted to begin as soon as he got back to Harvard. He and Alpert were trained clinicians, but this was not going to be like other drug tests. They were going to change the world.

"We're going to take a whole new approach with this research," Leary told Alpert. "Everyone thinks these drugs cause psychosis, but that's because they've been controlled by psychiatrists. Of course they're going to view this as psychosis. That's all they know. But there is really something deeper going on here, Richard. Wait until you try them. I learned more about psychology from these mushrooms than I did in graduate school. These drugs can revolutionize the way we conceptualize ourselves—not to mention the rest of the world. It'll be great. We'll give them to philosophers, poets, and musicians."

Alpert had been working with Leary for about a year at Harvard. Richard might have had the bigger office at the Department of Social Relations, but Tim was clearly the mentor in their relationship. There were about ten research psychologists in the department, all of them interested in the dynamics of the human personality. As he got to know Leary, Alpert started changing the way he looked at Harvard, and the way he looked at himself. Until Tim showed up, Richard was happily playing the professor role. He'd go to faculty meetings, sit in big chairs, and have tea from a silver tea service. It was easy to let the whole experience go to your head. Alpert would walk through Harvard Yard and begin to think he really *was* somebody. He was a member of the Harvard faculty. But Tim wasn't like that. He was the first guy Alpert ever met who was not impressed by Harvard. It was just a job.

Their relationship went beyond the office—even before they made the psychedelic bond. Tim arrived at Harvard with two children and no wife. Richard started hanging out with the kids, Susan and Jack, and began taking care of them. They started calling him "Uncle Dick," and he started acting out the role of surrogate mother. Richard was a bachelor. Tim was a bachelor with kids. Sometimes they'd find another baby sitter and go out drinking in Harvard Square. Lots of drinking, as in that 1950s kind of drinking.


Alpert had missed out on the mushrooms in Mexico and wasn't in Cambridge in the fall of 1960, when Leary started gathering together the tribe that would become the Harvard Psilocybin Project. Alpert had been teaching that semester as a visiting scholar at the University of California at Berkeley, but he was getting lots of fascinating reports about what was happening back at Harvard. He couldn't wait to get back and join the party, and his chance finally came one day in February 1961.

Alpert returned just as the biggest storm of the season dumped two feet of snow on the streets of Newton. Leary invited him over to his house for a Saturday-night initiation. By now, Leary and his growing band of graduate students had started experimenting with a new batch of drugs they'd gotten from Sandoz Laboratories in Switzerland. The drug was a synthesized form of psilocybin, the active ingredient in the magic mushrooms of Mexico. The psychic effects were the same, but the dose was easier to control.

While Alpert had been in California, Leary had begun to assemble an eclectic squadron of test pilots at his increasingly chaotic home. They included Beat poet Allen Ginsberg; jazz trumpeter Maynard Ferguson; William Burroughs, the legendary novelist and heroin addict; and Alan Watts, the popular Buddhist writer and commentator. Ginsberg was sitting at Leary's kitchen table the day Alpert burst in from the cold. Alpert joined them at the table, upon which stood a bottle of pink pills from Sandoz labs. He measured out ten milligrams of the drug and washed the pills down with a few gulps of beer.

Allen and Tim and Richard sat down in the kitchen and waited. Right away there was a bit of a melodrama. Tim's son, Jack, was upstairs when the boy's dog ran out of the house. The dog had been out galloping around in deep snow and came in panting heavily. They all started thinking, "Oh, no! The dog is dying!" Then they figured out that they really couldn't tell if the dog was dying because they were so high. Their thinking and senses were too distorted. Jack was eleven years old. He was upstairs watching television and a bit peeved that these silly adults were bothering him. He came down, assured them that the dog was fine, then marched back upstairs to the TV.

Alpert started really coming onto the psilocybin. There was too much talking in the kitchen, so he walked into the living room, a darker and more peaceful setting. He sat down on the sofa and tried to collect himself. Looking up, he saw some people over in the corner. *Who were they? Were they real?* Then he started to see them as images of himself in his various roles. They were hallucinations, but they seemed so real. There was the professor with a cap and gown. There was a pilot with a pilot's hat. There was the lover. At first, he was a bit amused by the vision. *Those are just my roles. That role can go. That role can go. I've had it with that role.* Then he saw himself as his father's son. The feeling changed. Wait a minute. *This drug is giving me amnesia! I'll wake up and I won't know who I am!* That was terrifying, but Alpert reminded himself that those roles weren't really important. *Stop worrying. It's fine. At least I have a body.* Then Alpert looked down on the couch at his body. *There's no body! Where's my body? There's no-body. There's nobody.* That was terrifying. He started to call out for Tim. *Wait a minute. How can I call out to Tim? Who was going to call for Tim? The minder of the store, me, would be calling for Tim. But who is me?* It was terrifying at first, but all of a sudden Alpert started watching the whole show with a kind of calm compassion.

At that moment, Richard Alpert met his own soul, his true soul. He jumped off the couch, ran out the door, and rolled down a snow-covered hill behind Leary's house. It was bliss. Pure bliss.

At the time, Alpert's parents were also living in Newton. Their home was just five blocks from Leary's house on Homer Street. It was three in the morning, but that didn't stop a stoned Richard Alpert from storming through the snow to go see his parents. When he got to his parents' house, he saw that no one had shoveled the deep snow off their walkway. So he went into the garage and got the shovel. In his drugged state, he saw himself as a young buck coming to the rescue. He was all-powerful. He would save his parents! It all seemed so mythological. Then he looked up at the window and saw his parents standing there. They were obviously peeved, or at least confused. Then they assumed that their son must have been drinking with Leary. Alpert saw them up in the window and waved at his startled parents. Then he stuck the shovel in the snow and started dancing around it. He felt so fine, perfectly fine.

Alpert recounts this tale of snowy bliss just a few days shy of the forty-seventh anniversary of the event, yet he remembers it like it was last night. As he tells the tale he's sitting beside a large picture window overlooking the rugged coast on the island of Maui. He says he's come here to Hawaii to die. But when he tells the story of that wondrous winter night his eyes light up like those of an excited little boy. He was twenty-nine years old then. He's seventy-six years old now. Leary is dead. Ginsberg is dead. Alpert is no longer a young buck. A nearly fatal stroke a decade earlier has left him paralyzed on his left side and confined to a wheelchair. The stroke nearly destroyed his ability to find words and speak them. He struggles mightily to tell the story, once again, of the events that changed his life.

"Until that moment I was always trying to be the good boy, looking at myself through other people's eyes," he says. "What did the mothers, fathers, teachers, colleagues want me to be? That night, for the first time, I felt good inside. It was OK to be me."

Healer
Cambridge, Massachusetts
Fall 1960

Andy Weil and Ronnie Winston were friends and dorm mates in Claverly Hall. They were both incoming Harvard freshmen when they walked into Leary's office on Divinity Lane and volunteered to be research subjects in his psychedelic research project. Weil had grown up in a middle-class family. Winston was the son of Harry Winston, the wealthy diamond and jewelry manufacturer whose creations hung around the necks of trophy wives and Hollywood starlets from coast to coast. Neither of them would officially take part in the project, but they would both play an important, little-known role in the rise and fall of Richard Alpert and Timothy Leary.

Winston would eventually be brought into the psychedelic family. Weil would not, and the implications of that unequal treatment would forever alter the careers and life paths of Timothy Leary and Richard Alpert.

Weil and Winston had both read *The Doors of Perception,* Huxley's book about the insights the British writer gleaned from his 1953 mescaline trip. They walked into Leary's little office on Divinity Avenue eager to fly off on their own mystical journey. They were a bit nervous when they sat down, but Leary soon put them at ease with his soft-spoken charm.

"Yes," Leary said, "Huxley was the trailblazer. You know, I didn't have a clue as to the potential of this research until I had my own experience with psilocybin mushrooms over the summer. At its core, you have to understand that this is not an intellectual exercise. It is experiential. It is, and I'm almost embarrassed to say it, religious. But it is more than religious. It is exhilarating. It shows us that the human brain possesses infinite potentialities. It can operate in space-time dimensions that we never dreamed even existed. I feel like I've awakened from a long ontological sleep."

Weil and Winston were on the edge of their seats.

"Anyway," Leary continued, "the research is pretty straightforward. Our subjects take a controlled dose of synthesized psilocybin. We make sure they are in a safe and comfortable setting. We're trying to get people from all walks of life, not just graduate students. We're giving this stuff to priests and prisoners and everyone in between. They do a session about once a month and are expected to write up a two- to three-page report describing the experience. Between sessions, we get together and discuss whatever insights we've gleaned from all this. Now, I assume neither of you have had any experience with these substances."

"No, sir, we have not," Weil replied. "But we are ready, willing, and able."

"I can see that," Leary said. "But I think we may have a little problem. How old are you boys?"

"Eighteen."

"That's what I was afraid of. You see, our agreement with the university does not allow us to use undergraduates in this research."

"That's what we were afraid of," Weil said. "To tell you the truth, some of us over at Claverly were thinking of running our own series of tests, and we were wondering if you could clue us in on how we might obtain some of these pills."

"Well, I could, but I'd better not do that, boys," Leary replied. "But if you're persistent, I'm sure you can find your own source."

Weil met separately with Professor Alpert. The answer was still the same. No, he could *not* participate in the experiments at the

Center for Personality Research. They had made an agreement with the university not to use undergraduate subjects in their research. To Weil, the meeting with Alpert had a very different feel than the get-together with Leary. Weil found Alpert uncomfortable to be around. Leary was a charmer. He was easygoing. Alpert was intense. He seemed too wrapped up in the role of the Harvard professor.

Weil and Winston were persistent. They weren't able to obtain their own psilocybin pills, but they did manage to get a supply of mescaline, a psychedelic drug synthesized from the peyote cactus. Weil wrote to Huxley, who suggested they try a company called Delta Chemical. Weil obtained some Harvard stationery and got to work. He couldn't fool the folks at Delta, who required too much official paperwork, but Weil found another company with looser drug-procurement procedures.

Once they got the drugs, Weil, Winston, and some other undergraduates started their own experiments in Claverly Hall. They were basically doing the same thing Leary was doing over at the Center for Personality Research. They'd take the drugs and write up reports about their experiences. Then they'd sit around and discuss them. Weil emerged as a leader of the little drug ring operating out of Claverly Hall. He collected about thirty reports on undergraduate mescaline trips. He didn't see the experiences as just an excuse to get high. He wasn't rebelling against anything. He was just curious, eager to understand what was going on inside his own brain.

Not much happened the first time he took mescaline. He was apprehensive. He'd later see that he was unconsciously resisting the drug. He didn't feel much of anything, and that disappointed him. He'd wanted to experience all the visual images he'd read about in those wild accounts of other mescaline eaters. That's what really fascinated him, but he didn't get any of that. On his second trip, he did have a more powerful emotional experience. Not hallucinations, but a kind of spiritual transcendence. It was a kind of serene feeling of connection with something higher. Everything just felt right—like he was seeing into the essence of things. But there was also something frightening about the experience. Andy was reluctant to just go with the flow. He didn't dare up the dose and go deeper. He could see that having any more of these insights might convince him that Harvard was a complete waste of time.

Weil was a calculating, ambitious young man. He had the next ten years of his life all mapped out. He'd later see that he'd somehow put the psychedelic experience in a box. He stopped experimenting with drugs. If he hadn't, he might have dropped out of school. Who knows what would have happened to him?

Meanwhile, Ronnie Winston had begun his own adventure with Richard Alpert. They'd met at a party. Ronnie was there with a girl Alpert knew, and the student and the professor started talking. Alpert invited Ronnie out to lunch, then for a ride in his airplane. They both came from wealthy East Coast families and had much in common. Alpert became infatuated with the young student. Ronnie was a brilliant, romantic-looking figure. He drove a Jaguar. He was a liberal arts student but had this idea for a project over at MIT involving solid rocket fuel. They didn't have sex, but they developed a kind of intimate friendship. Alpert shared some of his psilocybin with Winston. In Alpert's mind, Ronnie was a social friend—not a research subject—so he wasn't violating his agreement to keep undergraduates out of the psilocybin project.

Ronnie had made it into the inner circle around Leary and Alpert. Andy had not. At one point, Leary and Alpert had a conversation about Andy Weil. They didn't trust him. Alpert didn't like him. He was up to something. He had another agenda. They noticed that Weil had started covering the arts for the *Harvard Crimson,* the school newspaper. Maybe that was it. Maybe Weil was trying to infiltrate the project and write an exposé.

Weil saw a double standard in Alpert's embrace of Ronnie Winston. It was obvious that *some* undergraduates—and not just Ronnie—were being brought into the fold. Why not Andy? What was wrong with him? Ronnie had been a good friend. He'd even been Weil's guide during their mescaline sessions in Claverly Hall.

But that friendship ended when Winston started hanging out with Alpert.

Weil would find a way to get back at Richard Alpert and, in the process, put an end to his relationship with Ronnie Winston. Weil was determined to bring down the Harvard Psilocybin Project, and he would take on the assignment with the zeal of a jilted lover.

# CHAPTER THREE

# Sinners and Saints

Trickster
Concord State Prison
March 1961

Timothy Leary had a foreboding feeling the first time he entered the cage, through the imposing metal doors, and into the cell block. His surroundings seemed both strange *and* familiar. This time he was just visiting. He was a Harvard researcher with revolutionary ideas about how to reform the American prison system. By the end of the decade, Leary would walk into another prison and find the cell door slammed behind him. By then, he would be a real revolutionary, the guy Richard Nixon would call "the most dangerous man in America."

In the spring of 1961, Leary started calling the Harvard Psilocybin Project the "Harvard Psychedelic Project," and the research was in full swing. There were some interesting results. They'd given psychedelic drugs to some two hundred subjects—graduate students and faculty members from Harvard and MIT. Huston Smith had survived his New Year's Day trip. Dick Alpert had his night of snowy bliss. The vast majority of the other subjects reported that the sessions were among the most powerful, educational, and enlightening experiences of their lives. But Leary was a scientist, not a therapist. His job was to show that these drugs could benefit society. They needed a population they could accurately measure. What better place to go than into a prison system plagued with a history of rehabilitative failure—where some 70 percent of released inmates soon found themselves back behind bars. "What a boon to society—converting violent criminals to law-abiding citizens," Leary told a friend. "If we could teach the most unregenerate how to wash their own brains, then it would be a cinch to coach non-criminals to change their lives for the better."

Two years later, when the Harvard administration decided it was time for Leary and Alpert to move on, the embattled duo would cite two research projects in their failed bid to justify their academic existence—the Concord Prison Project and the Good Friday Experiment. The prison research sought to show how drug-induced insight could lower recidivism rates. The Good Friday subjects were to demonstrate that psychedelic drugs could produce genuine experiences of religious mysticism. Leary and Alpert would argue—unsuccessfully—that they had done research on the best and the baddest, on the saints and the sinners of American society.

By the summer of 1963, a more powerful drug, LSD (lysergic acid diethylamide), would replace psilocybin as the preferred chemical compound in Leary and Alpert's crusade to turn on a sleepy nation. It was a much stronger—and more dangerous—drug. And while they would become the most infamous psychedelic drug researchers in North America, they were by no means the first scientists to explore these realms.

LSD's bizarre effects on the human mind had been discovered two decades earlier when its inventor, Dr. Albert Hofmann, of the Sandoz Laboratories in Basel, Switzerland, became dizzy and had to stop working after accidentally dosing himself. The Swiss chemist had first synthesized the drug on November 16, 1938, while doing research on medical uses of ergot, a fungus that grows on rye bread. But Hofmann had put it on the shelf and forgotten about it until the spring of 1944. Hofmann had the world's first intentional LSD trip late in the afternoon of April 19, three days after getting the accidental dose. About fifty minutes after taking the drug, the chemist scribbled in his notebook what he was feeling in his mind, reporting "slight dizziness, unrest, difficulty in concentration, visual disturbances, marked desire to laugh." Hofmann was soon too stoned to write. He asked his assistant to accompany him home. They rode bikes from the lab to Hofmann's house, a trip that would be forever remembered in the annals of psychedelic history. "My field of vision swayed before me," Hofmann would later write. "Objects appeared distorted like the images in curved mirrors. I had the impression of being unable to move from the spot, although my assistant told me afterwards that we had cycled at a good pace."

His condition only worsened once he got home:

*The faces of those present appeared like grotesque colored masks; strong agitation alternating with paresis; the head, body and extremities sometimes cold and numb, a metallic taste on the tongue; throat dry and shrilled; a feeling of suffocation; confusion alternating with a clear appreciation of the situation.*

*I lost all control of time; space and time became more and more disorganized and I was overcome with fear that I was going crazy. The worst part of it was that I was clearly aware of my condition though I was incapable of stopping it. Occasionally I felt as being outside my body. I thought I had died. My "Ego" was suspended somewhere in space and I saw my body lying dead on the sofa. I observed and registered clearly that my "alter ego" was moving around the room, moaning.*

It was an amazing journey, but what was equally amazing to Hofmann was that he experienced all this with such a tiny—0.25 mg—dose of LSD. This new drug was two to three thousand times stronger than mescaline, which scientists once thought to be the most powerful chemical agent available to alter the human mind. All of Leary and Alpert's early research was done with psilocybin, the drug that put the magic in those Mexican mushrooms, and mescaline, which is found naturally in the peyote cactus. Leary didn't even try LSD until December 1961, eighteen months after his first mushroom trip at the villa in Cuernavaca.

*Psychedelic,* the word used to describe the experience one has on mescaline, psilocybin, and LSD, was just coming into popular use in the early 1960s. Huxley and the man who turned him on, the English psychiatrist Humphrey Osmond, invented the word. Osmond had begun experimenting with psychedelics in the early 1950s, first with mescaline in England and then more systematically with LSD at Weyburn Mental Hospital in Saskatchewan, where he received funding for his research from the Canadian government and the Rockefeller Foundation. Osmond's studies came to the attention of Huxley, who wrote the psychiatrist in the winter of 1953 and invited him to come by for a visit if he ever found himself in Los Angeles. Huxley was even kind enough to include a signed copy of his newest book, *The Devils of Loudun,* a nonfiction account of demonic possession and religious fanaticism in seventeenth-century France. Los Angeles seemed a world away from Osmond's remote Saskatchewan home, but three months later he was invited to deliver a paper at the American Psychiatric Association convention in Los Angeles. He wrote back to Huxley telling him that, as chance would have it, he would soon be in southern California.

Huxley was at the breakfast table with his wife, Maria, the morning Osmond's letter arrived.

"Why don't we invite the chap to stay with us," Aldous suggested.

"Aldous, you don't like having people stay here. You don't even like it when Julian stays here," Maria replied, referring to the novelist's famous brother, the biologist Sir Julian Huxley.

For some reason, Huxley insisted on having someone he'd never met stay at their home, extending that invitation to Osmond by return post.

Osmond was surprised at Huxley's generosity but told his wife he thought it would be better not to impose on the famous couple. He'd be more comfortable just staying at the convention hotel.

"Do what you want," Jane Osmond replied. "But if you do, you'll never forgive yourself."

Jane was right. Osmond wound up staying at the Huxley home and serving as the guide for a mescaline trip that would be immortalized in Huxley's next book, *The Doors of Perception*.

Huxley's 1953 mescaline trip revealed many things, including the limitations of using the word *psychotomimetic* to describe his experience. Yes, these drugs could mimic the psychotic state. They could give the user feelings of paranoia. But they could also promote positive insight. They could reveal mystical realms. "Aldous and I decided that the words we were using for these strange chemical instruments were idiotic," Osmond later recalled. "We wanted to encourage people to use them intelligently."

Another researcher had begun using the word *fantastica* to describe the psychedelic experience. That was a fun word, Osmond and Huxley agreed, but it kind of begged the question. It biased the user to expect something strange and bizarre—based in fantasy. You could call these drugs *hallucinogens*, but not everyone who took them actually had hallucinations, and even if they did, that seemed to place a negative connotation on the visions and insight that could be obtained from the drugs. They needed a more neutral term.

Huxley and Osmond exchanged a series of letters in which they suggested various words to describe these powerful drugs, sometimes composing a little rhyme to try them out in a creative context. Huxley suggested *phanerothyme*, which meant "to make the soul visible," along with the poem:

> *To make this trivial world sublime*
> *Take half a gramme of phanerothyme.*

Not bad, Osmond thought, but not quite right. It sounded a bit too botanical. Osmond had a little guide of Latin terms that was designed for use by medical students. Consulting that reference book, he decided that *psyche* was more neutral than *psycho,* and then he came across the word *delos,* "to reveal." There it was. *Psychedelic* would be the word, and Osmond's little poem sealed the deal:

> *To fathom hell or soar angelic*
> *Just take a pinch of psychedelic.*

Humphrey Osmond was also the author of a much-discussed study in the 1950s that reported some success in treating alcoholics with LSD. Osmond initially thought the drug produced symptoms similar to delirium tremens. Producing a terrifying artificial delirium might frighten an alcoholic into change. Between 1954 and 1960, Osmond and his colleagues treated some two thousand alcoholics under carefully controlled conditions and came to see that it was insight, not terror, that seemed to help these drunks reform.

It was this research that would briefly bring Bill Wilson, a co-founder of Alcoholics Anonymous, into the early psychedelic scene. Wilson was—like Huston Smith—a big fan of Gerald Heard. "Bill W.," as he is known to his AA minions, was a hard-drinking businessman who got sober in the 1930s with the help of an evangelical Christian movement known as the Oxford Group. He was the primary author of the so-called Big Book, the classic self-help volume that outlines AA's twelve-step program for sober living and spiritual recovery. Wilson was clearly influenced by the evangelical movement, but he was also a somewhat eclectic spiritual seeker; this inclination can be seen in the twelve-step program's emphasis on alcoholics turning to a self-defined "higher power," to God "*as we understood Him.*"

In August 1956, one year after Wilson turned over the AA leadership to an elected board of directors, Heard guided Wilson on an LSD trip that would have a profound impact on the world's best-known recovering alcoholic. Wilson took what was probably his first LSD trip at the Los Angeles Veterans Administration Hospital on August 29, 1956. According to notes taken by Heard, the founder of AA felt "an enormous enlargement," and his insights included the realization that "people shouldn't take themselves so damn seriously." Shortly after that acid trip, Huston Smith accompanied Heard on a trip to Kansas City and spent two hours in a hotel room listening to Wilson and Heard talk about the acid trip. Wilson was blown away by the drug and said the experience was a dead ringer for the famous night in the 1930s when he fell down on his knees and had an epiphany about founding his twelve-step program.

One of the main tenets of the group's recovery program is that alcoholics and other drug addicts must go through some kind of spiritual awakening to overcome their addiction. Wilson thought an LSD trip could be an effective tool for AA members who had little interest—or negative feelings—about religion and spirituality. The founder of Alcoholics Anonymous had several LSD sessions in the mid-1950s, including one with researchers working with Dr. Sidney Cohen at UCLA. Wilson had a group drug session with Tom Powers, a close Wilson associate who handled public relations for AA. Cohen had proposed a low-dose session with the two AA leaders, but he made the mistake of giving Wilson another option.

"Well, there are more pills available should you want them," Cohen said.

"Don't ever tell that to a drunk," said Wilson, who insisted on taking a double dose.

Bill Wilson would have another cameo appearance in the psychedelic story. In a letter to Timothy Leary dated July 17, 1961, Wilson wrote that Huxley had "referred enthusiastically to your work." Wilson goes on to write that "though LSD and some kindred alkaloids have had an amazingly bad press, there seems no doubt of their immense and growing value." The AA founder also hints that he knew of Leary's own problems with alcohol, adding that Tim might "find some interest in Alcoholics Anonymous—its principles and mechanism."

It was Humphrey Osmond's research that originally inspired Wilson to try LSD. "Early on I told Bill this was good news," Osmond said, "but he was far from pleased with the idea of alcoholics being assailed by some strange chemical. But later on Bill got extremely interested. He likened his experience to his original AA vision of seeing this chain of drunks around the world. This caused quite a scandal in Alcoholics Anonymous. They became very ambivalent about their great founder, even though they wouldn't have existed if he hadn't had an adventurous kind of mind."


Osmond's work also intrigued another American with an adventurous kind of mind—Timothy Leary. If Osmond was able to help alcoholics break their patterns of destructive behavior, why not try psychedelic drugs on hardened criminals? Leary invited two administrators from the Massachusetts Correctional Institute at Concord to join him for lunch at the Harvard Faculty Club to discuss his ideas. Not wanting to scare them off with his gleaming white tennis shoes, Leary decided to switch into more conventional leather footwear. The shoes went unnoticed, and the meeting went well. These prison wardens would try anything—even mushroom pills—to reduce their recidivism rate. But Leary first had to get the support of the prison psychiatrist, which necessitated that first trip out to Concord Prison and that strange feeling that he'd been there before and would be there again. But Leary's mood lightened when he met the prison shrink. To his surprise, the guy was an African-American— the first black psychiatrist Leary had ever met. His name was Dr. Madison Presnell, and he and Leary really hit it off. Leary found Presnell gracefully hip. He had a twinkle in his eye and a wise, cool way about him. Here was a guy ready to try something new.

Once he got prison officials on board, Leary put together a group of Harvard graduate students to help interview prisoners, run the drug sessions, and monitor their progress. One of the first guys Leary turned to was Ralph Metzner, a German-born, twenty-six-year-old graduate student who'd gotten his bachelor's degree from Oxford University in England and had been awarded a scholarship to do his doctoral work at Harvard. Metzner was attracted to the Harvard Department of Social Relations because of the program's interdisciplinary approach—the way it brought together social psychology, clinical psychology, sociology, and cultural anthropology. Metzner had taken a seminar with Leary the semester before they started the mushroom project. Leary was working out a philosophy he called "Existential-Transactionalism," which built upon Eric Berne's writings on game theory. Berne would later write the best-selling book *I'm OK, You're OK.* In the early 1960s, Leary and Alpert were constantly talking about all the games people play. They were playing the "professor game." Students were playing the "student game."

Metzner was impressed with how Leary questioned the roles academics and psychologists play out in their work—something Leary was doing long before his first psychedelic experience. Metzner agreed with Leary that the usual relationships that psychologists have in their work, such as doctor-patient or experimenter-subject, are artificial, asymmetric power relationships. One person is always superior to the other person, by the nature of the relationship. Leary was looking for another way to relate to patients, and to people in general. If someone needs psychological help, why not just go to the guy's house, sit around the kitchen table, drink some coffee, and talk about it? Psychologists should present themselves as resources, not as doctors or authority figures. Metzner found Leary's method very egalitarian, and very refreshing.

Leary's approach to the prisoners who were to be his research subjects was equally egalitarian. It was not unusual for prisoners to act as guinea pigs in drug experiments, putting their own health at risk in the hopes of an early parole. Leary's approach was different. Magic mushrooms had given him a life-changing experience. He wanted to share that experience with the inmates. It was essential, Leary stressed, that the Harvard researchers actually take the drugs *with* the prisoners. *That* was the revolutionary approach, not the fact that the inmates were getting some experimental drug.

At the time, the star of the Harvard psychology department was B. F. Skinner, the famous behaviorist. Skinner had no interest in human "consciousness" and believed that the best way to understand human behavior was through the stimulus/response model.

Leary was going against the grain, and that was great news to Ralph Metzner. He and his fellow graduate students were sick and tired of sitting around plugging numbers into calculators. It seemed like all they did were boring statistical studies. And here was Leary, talking about *experiences,* very meaningful experiences. Metzner was ignorant, and a bit anxious, about taking the drug. But he was also intrigued by Leary's requirement that all his graduate students try out the drugs they would be giving to the prisoners. They were even encouraged to trip *with* the prisoners.

Leary wasn't sure if Metzner could handle himself in the rough-and-tumble of Concord Prison. Could he really deal with all those robbers, rapists, and murderers? Leary decided to take a chance with Metzner—betting that the determined young German could handle the psychedelic experience *and* the prison experience. So one cold day in early March, Metzner showed up at the doorstep of Leary's Newton home for his first test trip.

For Metzner, it was an experience of something he had never even imagined. Everywhere he looked he saw glowing jeweled objects. Ordinary people were instantly transformed into angels. At one point, he walked out into the snow to get some fresh air. There was some garbage by the back door, and he heard a voice tell him, "Don't look at the garbage." He experienced that random thought in a whole new way, seeing for the first time how his thoughts were preprogrammed. He didn't choose to have that thought. So where did these thoughts come from? Maybe he could direct his thoughts in other ways. Isn't that what psychotherapy was all about? We can stop thinking old habitual thoughts. The moment was a turning point, the beginning of a shift in the way Ralph Metzner looked at psychology, mysticism, and the mind.

Metzner's next trip was not as inspiring, at least not at first. But he would soon learn why and explain it all in *The Psychedelic Experience,* a book he would author with Leary and Alpert. One of the trio's key findings on the intelligent use of psychedelics would be the importance of "set and setting" in determining the outcome of a drug trip. The "set" is the mind-set, the expectations the user has about what is going to happen. The "setting" is the environment in which the effects of a given plant or chemical are to be experienced. One's setting should be comfortable—perhaps a dimly lit living room with large pillows and soothing music, or an open field full of spring wildflowers, or a cliff top at Big Sur. Certainly not a depressing prison hospital room with gray walls, a black asphalt floor, and bars on the windows. Certainly not a cell shared with a Polish embezzler and a heroin addict from Dorchester. Yet those two inmates were among the first volunteers to take the mushroom pills with Leary, Metzner, and Gunther Weil, another graduate student (no relation to Andrew Weil) who was helping conduct the prison research. Leary's idea was to give the subjects predrug personality tests, guide them through the psychedelic sessions, and then have them retested to see what kind of short-term changes had occurred in their outlook on life. The first two sessions were held on March 27, 1961, and brought the Harvard psychologists together with five Concord prisoners for an encounter that none of them would ever forget.

Metzner and two of the prisoners each took twenty milligrams of psilocybin from the prison psychiatrist, who was there to provide medical supervision. They all sat back and took in their bleak surroundings. There were four beds, a large table, and a few chairs. Leary brought along a record player, a tape recorder, and some books of classical art to try to soften the setting, but there wasn't much you could do to transform a prison infirmary into a serene setting.

Metzner started coming on to the drug. He stared at the gray wall before him. It was like a horror movie. All his fears were projected on the prison walls. It was like a newsreel of all the evil acts in human history. Metzner started sweating, moaning, and groaning. Then Gunther Weil came over and gently put his hand on Ralph and said, "How are you doing, man?" Suddenly, everything changed. Gunther was the mother of God, full of compassion, flowing with human kindness. The horror turned into compassion. All it took was a simple touch.

Metzner and the Harvard team spent nine months at the prison, running monthly psilocybin sessions for about a dozen convicts. In between the sessions, the convicts would sit through group therapy sessions and take personality tests. According to Leary's findings, these follow-up tests showed less depression and hostility, more responsibility and cooperation. More prisoners signed up for the experiment.

Meanwhile, news of the Harvard mushroom project was getting out to the larger academic community. When visitors came to Harvard to check out the research project, Leary often took them out to Concord Prison. Among those sitting down with the convicts were Gerald Heard, Aldous Huxley, and Alan Watts.

Follow-up programs worked with prisoners after they were released. Nearly two years later, in January 1963, Leary would claim that 75 percent of the turned-on prisoners who were released had stayed out of jail. He had cut the recidivism rate in half. He'd found a way to solve the nation's crime problem.

Prison officials were skeptical. This was no great breakthrough. If you shower this much personal attention on inmates before and after they are released, of course you cut the return rate. It had nothing to do with mushrooms. The biggest problem with the prison project was that there was no control group of prisoners who were given that kind of attention but no mushroom pills.

Even those working with Leary came to doubt the long-term success of the Concord Prison Project. Alpert believed that the basic therapeutic model was sound, but he thought Leary needed to stick with the project and conduct long-term studies. Metzner conceded that the researchers fell victim to "the halo effect," putting their findings in the best possible light. Even Leary admitted that it was hard to build upon the initial revelatory insights that he and his prison subjects shared after taking the mushroom pills. "In the sessions," he would later recall, "we were all gods, all men at once. We were all two-billion-year-old seed centers pulsing together. Then as time slowly froze we were reborn in the old costumes and picked up the tired games. We weren't yet ready to act on our revelation."

Teacher
Marsh Chapel, Boston University
Good Friday, 1962

Timothy Leary, Richard Alpert, and Ralph Metzner were amazed by the religious experiences they were having on psychedelic drugs, but they had no context to understand those feelings of wonder, awe, and connectedness. They were having mystical experiences, but they were not mystics. They were not priests, not even scholars of religion. They were clinical psychologists. What did *they* really know about shamanism or mysticism?

Enter Huston Smith.

Here was the member of the team who really knew something about the varieties of religious experience. Smith had already written the book on the great world religions. He had described those exotic faiths to the American public in the first public-television program to explore that territory. He had been practicing yoga for more than a decade. But even Huston Smith was not quite ready for what he was about to experience in Marsh Chapel on a fateful Friday in 1962.

It would go down in the annals of psychedelic history as the Good Friday Experiment. The project was the brainchild of Walter Pahnke, a medical doctor and Protestant minister who designed this research project for his PhD in Religion and Society at Harvard. Leary was his principal academic adviser. Twenty seminary students from nearby Andover Newton Theological Seminary were selected for a double-blind experiment in which half the seminarians were given capsules containing thirty milligrams of psilocybin and half were given an active placebo containing nicotinic acid, which induced a tingling sensation. Pahnke thought that might fool those students into thinking they had gotten the psychedelic drug. All twenty students were to gather in a small basement sanctuary at Marsh Chapel, across the Charles River from Harvard, on the Boston University campus. Upstairs, the Reverend

Howard Thurmond, a black clergyman who helped inspire the work of the Reverend Martin Luther King, delivered his Good Friday sermon to a congregation unaware of the experiment being conducted downstairs. Thurmond's sermon, the hymns, and other sounds from the service were piped down so the research subjects could follow along.

Pahnke was no typical Harvard student. He already had a medical degree when he arrived at the divinity school. He rode a bicycle with balloon tires, and pedaled around campus with fearsome energy. There was something strident in the way he pedaled up to a building, tossing his bike down and marching into class.

His Good Friday Experiment was trying to determine if psilocybin could produce an "authentic religious experience." Leary was not thrilled with Pahnke's protocol. He thought Pahnke himself should experience the effects of psychedelic drugs to truly understand what he was talking about, but Pahnke refused. Leary also knew that few of the students who got nicotinic acid would be fooled into thinking they had gotten psilocybin, and those who got the psychoactive drug would certainly know they had the real thing. Years later, when he returned to Harvard with Alpert to celebrate the twentieth anniversary of their ouster from the university, Leary would praise Pahnke's work but laugh at some of his presumptions. "It was probably the greatest Good Friday in two thousand years—or it was for half of the subjects. The control subjects got to sit there and read the Bible," Leary quipped. "If we learned one thing from that experience it was how foolish it was to use a double-blind experiment with psychedelics. After five minutes, no one's fooling anyone. We also learned that we all had to do the work together, with no principal investigator, because once you put that pill in your mouth, *you* are the principal investigator—like it or not."

Leary was right about the placebos. Once the psilocybin kicked in, it was clear who the real test pilots were in the basement of Marsh Chapel. The small underground room where the day's events unfolded has a low roof, giving it the feel of a tomb. The only natural light shines from three tiny stained-glass windows, including one depicting Jesus holding an open Bible. "And ye shall know the truth," it reads. "And the truth shall set you free." On that eventful Good Friday back in 1962, ten of the divinity students sat in their pews before the altar, politely following the readings and hymns that were being piped down from upstairs. Those who got the real thing were lying back on the pews, or on the floor. Others were wandering around murmuring prayers of wonderment. "God is everywhere," one cried out. "Oh, the Glory."

Huston Smith was one of the preselected guides for the Good Friday Experiment, none of whom knew in advance whether they would get the drug or the placebo. Huston got the drug. Until that day, Smith had never had a direct personal encounter with God, the kind of experience that Indian yogis and Pentecostal Christians talk about. Smith hadn't had that experience in his previous psychedelic sessions, as powerful as those trips had been, but this time was different. Maybe it was the Protestant worship service—a setting that fostered a deep connection with Smith's upbringing as a child of Methodist missionaries. Huston's mother had been a music teacher, and passed along her acute sensitivity to harmonic resonance. Upstairs in the main chapel, a soprano was delivering a solo. Listening to it piped downstairs—through the audio system and the prism of the mushroom pills—Smith knew this was no human voice he heard. It was the song of an angel. He would never forget the opening and closing verses of that consciousness-expanding hymn:

*My times are in Thy hand;*
*My God, I wish them there;*
*My life, my friends, my soul I leave*
*Entirely to Thy care.*

*My times are in Thy hand,*
*I'll always trust in Thee;*
*And after death, at Thy right hand*
*I shall forever be.*

That Good Friday service was a powerful, cosmic homecoming for Huston Smith, but the service commemorating Christ's crucifixion was not without its comic moments. One of the seminary students who'd gotten the drug escaped from the chapel and headed down Commonwealth Avenue, oblivious to Smith's pleas for him to return to the church. Huston would later learn that the student had become convinced that God had chosen him to announce the dawning of the Messianic Age—that the world was about to experience one thousand years of universal peace. To the passersby on Commonwealth Avenue, he just looked like a guy zonked out of his mind. Huston ran after the student, who was heading toward the building that housed the Boston University School of Theology. When the student reached the front steps, he accosted a postman who was carrying a special-delivery letter for the dean of the school. The would-be messiah grabbed the letter out of the startled postman's hand and crumpled it up. There was nothing special about *this* delivery. *He* had the special delivery in his heart—and it was good news for the dean of theology and the rest of mankind. Huston managed to get the letter back by prying loose the crazed student's fingers. Then Huston and another of the guides overpowered the kid and dragged him back to the chapel. Pahnke gave the divine messenger a shot of Thorazine to settle him down.

Smith—still stoned on the psilocybin but able to snap out of it enough to attend to the escaping student—returned to the chapel and another rowdy scene. Ten of the subjects were enraptured, but the other half were feeling left out and disgruntled. They responded to the stoned students' profound utterances with derisive laughter and incredulous hoots. Smith himself turned to one of his colleagues, Paul Lee. Huston's eyes were wide with the wonder of it all. "It's true, isn't it?" Smith said, certain that his profound proclamation needed no elaboration. Lee had gotten the placebo and didn't have the slightest idea what the blissed-out philosophy professor was talking about, but decided to play along.

"Yeah, Huston. 'It' is true—whatever *it* is."

"It" was the religious outlook, God, and everything that flows from God's reality. And it was something Smith would keep with him for the rest of his life. His encounter that Good Friday was the most powerful experience he would ever have of God's personal nature. Sure, he always *believed* that God was love, that God loves him and he loves God, but he had never *experienced* that love in such a profound and personal way. From that moment on, he knew that life is a miracle, every moment of it, and that the only appropriate way to respond and be mindful of that gift of God's love was to share it with the rest of the world. It wasn't all that different from the message of the would-be messiah. Huston was just a bit more contained in his delivery.

Rather than instant enlightenment, however, Paul Lee got a severe case of prickly heat courtesy of the nicotine acid that was supposed to fool him into thinking he got the drug. Lee was not fooled. He'd already had his first psychedelic trip, and he knew what he was missing. He was one of the guys laughing at the stoned divinity students, especially the one who went up to the piano and started giving a sermon about his beatific vision.

Lee knew something about Christian theology. At the time, he was working as the teaching assistant to Paul Tillich, the great German-born theologian who taught at Harvard Divinity School from 1954 to 1962. To the sober Lee, there was nothing profound about the silly scene unfolding in Marsh Chapel. "It was the stupidest thing you ever saw in your life," he later told a friend. "Guys were crawling around you on the floor on their hands and knees."


Paul Lee had been brought into the circle by Huston Smith, who'd invited him over to his house one day for a meeting with Timothy Leary.

"Tim is looking to get some people from the divinity school," Huston told him. "They want to turn around the psychologists' understanding of these substances. They want to replace the psychotic model with a mystical model, but these guys don't know beans about mysticism."

Leary was particularly intent on recruiting Harvard theologians and divinity students as research subjects for his drug tests. Among those he approached was Harvey Cox, who was studying at Harvard Divinity School.

"We're working with these inmates over at Concord Prison, and they keep coming up with all this religious imagery," he told Cox. "Some are seeing hell. Others are having all sorts of beatific visions."

Cox would go on in 1965 to publish *The Secular City,* an international best seller that made him one of the best-known theological voices of the 1960s and 1970s. He almost signed up but changed his mind at the last minute, unsure that he was psychologically prepared for a quick trip to heaven or hell.

Alpert and Leary even tried to turn on Paul Tillich, a theologian best known for his description of God as "the ground of being." They ran into him one morning at a restaurant. They went over to the great man, introduced themselves, and began describing their research. Tillich—the absolute paragon of the German theology professor—was not impressed.

"Do you really think that *this* is for someone like me? Someone who grew up in a medieval town where my father was the minister—a walled German town with all its culture? Do you really think all that tradition can be found in the form of a pill?"

"Yeah! Yeah! We think it can," Alpert exclaimed.

"Yes, sir," Leary added. "That is now the case."

Like Harvey Cox, Professor Tillich politely passed on the psychedelic invitation. But Paul Lee took the bait.

Lee's first trip was on a Saturday evening at Leary's house. Leary couldn't make the session, so he sent one of his graduate students over to administer the psychedelic sacrament. It was quite a production. Someone put Wagner's "Flight of the Valkyries" on the record player. *Dum-da-da-da-dum. Dum-da-da-da-dum. Dum-DA-DA-DA-dum. Dum-da-da-da.* Someone vomited. Then the fireplace backed up and filled up with smoke. At one point, a grad student who was also tripping started making aggressive moves toward his wife, pretending to smash her skull with his fist, pounding it into the pillow next to her head. They managed to quiet him down, and after an hour or two things settled into a more spiritual mood.

It was the height of the Cold War, and everyone was thinking about the Russians and the bomb. For Paul Lee, the psychedelic journey felt like an atomic bomb going off in his mind. Your structured rationality exploded. The experience fascinated him. It was so intense, and then it would be over, and he couldn't remember exactly what had happened. Things seemed to happen in an instant, but then he'd see that hours had actually gone by. His sense of time seemed so distorted on the drugs, or maybe it was his normal sense that was distorted. On the drugs, it seemed like the eternal now. It was amazing, but it was also frightening—kind of like jumping out of an airplane.

All of the subjects in the Good Friday Experiment—including the control group, the one that got the placebo—completed questionnaires designed to determine whether they had a mystical experience. The survey asked them to what extent they experienced a sense of unity, transcendence of time and space, a sense of sacredness, a sense of objective reality, a deeply felt positive mood, ineffability, paradoxicality, and transiency. Pahnke reported that "eight out of ten of the experimental subjects experienced at least seven out of the nine categories. None of the control group, when each individual was compared to his matched partner, had a score which was higher."

Pahnke's research was later cited in a story in *Time* magazine, which effusively reported that "all students who had taken the drug psilocybin experienced a mystical consciousness that resembled those described by saints and ascetics." *Time*'s rave review, titled "Mysticism in the Lab," was published as a debate was raging in the United States over to what extent LSD and other psychedelic drugs should be criminalized. The forces of criminalization won, and LSD was outlawed in October 1966.

Twenty years later, psychedelic drug researcher Rick Doblin spent three years tracking down and interviewing sixteen of the twenty students who gathered for that Good Friday service in Marsh Chapel. Half of the seminarians—five who got psilocybin and five from the control group—were currently working as ministers. Others went into such professions as stockbroker, lawyer, community developer, social worker, administrative assistant, and educator. Nearly all of them were married, and all were working and self-supporting. And all but two welcomed the chance to reflect on what happened to them on that memorable day in the spring of 1962.

Here's one recollection:

> *I was kneeling there praying and beginning to feel like I was experiencing the kind of prayer life that I experienced back when I was in the seventh grade, eleven or twelve years old. It was the kind of experiences that you knew that something great was happening. I started to go to the root of all being, and discovered that . . . you never quite get there. That was my discovery during that time. . . . It's a philosophy and a theology that I hold yet today. You can approach the fullness of all being in either prayer, or in the psilocybin experience. You can reach out, but you can't dive down . . . and hit that root.*
>
> *The discovery within that experience is that you could approach God by two different ways. You either get to the root, the ground of all being, or the fullness of all being. And in getting to the root, you'll strive, you'll come closer and closer, but it's always half, and you'll think another half step, another half step, and you'll never quite get there. The fullness, to approach the fullness of God, is the only way to approach God.*

Another student—not the one chased down Commonwealth Avenue by Huston Smith—tried to leave the chapel. His mushroom trip was not an entirely positive experience:

*Shortly after receiving the capsule, all of a sudden I just wanted to laugh. I began to go into a very strong paranoid experience. And I found it to be scary. The chapel was dark and I hated it in there, just absolutely hated it in there. And I got up and left. I walked down the corridor and there was a guard, a person stationed at the door so individuals wouldn't go out, and he says, "Don't go outside," and I said, "Oh no, I won't. I'll just look outdoors." And I went to the door and out I went. They sent [a group leader] out after me. We went back into the building and again, I hated to be in that building and being confined because there were bars on the window and I felt literally like I was in prison. One of the things that was probably happening to me was a reluctance to just flow. I tried to resist that and as soon as resistance sets in there's likely to be conflict and there's likely, I think, for there to be anxiety.*

---

Decades after the gathering in Marsh Chapel, Huston Smith and Timothy Leary also looked back at the long-term lessons from the Good Friday Experiment. The way each remembers the event says volumes about the difference between these two members of the Harvard Psychedelic Club. For Smith, the memory was one of profound gratitude to Walter Pahnke, who died nine years later in a scuba-diving accident. Smith recalls the experiment as a profound revelation that forever changed the way he saw God, himself, and the rest of the world. For Smith, the Good Friday Experiment was about reconciliation.

For Leary, it was different. Timothy Leary was not a reconciler. He was a rebel. In his account of the Good Friday Experiment, Leary remembers how difficult it was for Pahnke to get permission and funding for follow-up research (difficulties that no doubt stemmed from his close association with the rebel psychologist from Harvard). Smith saw the love of God on Good Friday. Leary saw something more sinister in Pahnke's subsequent problems getting support for his research.

"We remembered Huxley's observation that the original sin was the ingestion of a brain-change fruit in the Garden," Leary wrote in his autobiography. "There was not much chance that the bureaucrats of Christian America were going to accept our research results, no matter how objective.

"We had run up against the Judeo-Christian commitment to one God, one religion, one reality that has cursed Europe for centuries and America since our founding days. Drugs that open the mind to multiple realities inevitably lead to a polytheistic view of the universe. We sensed that the time for a new humanist religion based on intelligent good-natured pluralism and scientific paganism had arrived."

Leary was infamous for such pronouncements, and his rebel spirit helped set the tone for the counterculture of the 1960s. But those who worked closely with the man caution against oversimplifying his significance. He was more than just a rebel trying to bring down "the system." Metzner suggests the word *trickster* as the best way to describe Timothy Leary.

"In American Indian lore, the trickster is a teacher who uses jokes and trickery to get people to wake up," Metzner said. "They don't give you advice like a benevolent guru. They don't want you to give up your own responsibility. Tim was provocative. He was trying to get you to think for yourself—and have fun. Take it lightly. That was part of the Irish in him. He was a rascal. A satirist. He had razor-sharp insight. He didn't mind being provocative in his language, and he didn't bother to correct anybody's misconception of him. But basically, he was a very positive person, one of the most genial and incredibly intelligent people I ever met."

Another leader in the "LSD cult" of the 1960s, Art Kleps, remembers Leary as a man with awesome charm: "His voice trilled and tinkled, caressing the ear with gentle melodies and punctuations. . . . He almost never raised it. Even when angry or malicious, the voice stayed within the limits of its charm. . . . His voice, as if it had some separate spirit or function of its own, did not, like most voices, simply carry Tim's thoughts like a load in a cart; it often spoofed and laughed at what it was required to support, thereby anticipating and disarming the critical reactions of his audience. Much of Tim's wit relied on these disarming vocal nuances; it does not come through as well in his written words." Like Metzner, Kleps saw the trickster in Leary. "Many thought Tim was spoofing when he wasn't, or thought he wasn't when he was. Tim's playfulness had no consistency, no foundation in logical analysis or a stable set of values. It was simply employed to take the edge off, to provide an escape hatch, to disarm."

Harvey Cox, the Harvard divinity student who declined Leary's offer to try psychedelic drugs, has another take on the infamous psychology professor. "Later on I did experiment with psychedelics," Cox said. "For a while I continued to think LSD had great promise—if it had been used in a controlled and careful way. But Leary was such an egotistical guy. He saw himself as forging new rules for psychological research and questioning the assumptions of the academy, eventually making himself the messiah for spiritual discovery."

Cox knew all four members of the Harvard Psychedelic Club and thinks Huston Smith had the most lasting positive impact on society. "Huston was one of the pioneers in how to understand world religions while remaining rooted in your own tradition," Cox said. "He was a Christian. He never really let go of that, and showed us how having a real rooted spirituality of your own can help you understand these other traditions even better. That has come to be the currency of interfaith movement and religious studies today. All of us who teach religious studies today are more heavily into comparative religion. You have to be. This is a world of religious pluralism. You have to see what can be learned from other religious traditions, and how that can enrich your perspective. That's the model we use now at Harvard Divinity School."

Another informed perspective comes from Walter Houston Clark, a professor of the psychology of religion at Andover Newton Theological Seminary and one of the men involved in the Good Friday Experiment. He notes that Leary was a lapsed Catholic and in the eyes of many Christians would be considered a "sinner." Clark suggests that *saint,* at least as William James defines the word, may be a better label for Timothy Leary. In *The Varieties of Religious Experience,* James speaks of saints having "a feeling of being in a wider life than that of this world's selfish interests; and a conviction, not merely intellectual, but as it were sensible, of an Ideal Power."

Leary was uninterested in the worldly prestige of a Berkeley or Harvard professorship. He saw tyranny in any man's efforts to impose standards of behavior upon him. In Clark's view, Leary most certainly had the sense of an "Ideal Power" in his life. His life after leaving Harvard would be an adventurous and sorrowful one, with multiple prison terms, a daughter's suicide, and a diagnosis of inoperable prostate cancer.

"Leary's equanimity, keenness of mind, his sense of humor, empathy and compassion under misfortunes, which could crush ordinary men, would be impossible were it not linked to some source of strength in that wider life James also connects with strength of soul. . . . All this is not to say that Timothy Leary is a second Jesus Christ, Socrates, or Francis of Assisi. He is only a first Timothy Leary. He is a human being who has made his share of mistakes," Clark wrote in *Chemical Ecstasy: Psychedelic Drugs and Religion,* a book published in 1969, seven years after the Good Friday Experiment. "Time will tell whether Timothy Leary is a pied piper or one of the perceptive prophets of the age."

# CHAPTER FOUR

# Crimson Tide

Healer
Cambridge, Massachusetts
May 1963

It was a heady time to be editor in chief of the *Harvard Crimson*. You sat in a chair into which the name of one of your predecessors, Franklin D. Roosevelt, class of 1904, was carved in wood. The White House was occupied by another Harvard man and former *Crimson* editor, John F. Kennedy, class of 1940. "If the *Crimson* didn't show up at the White House, we'd get calls from Schlesinger's office or Bundy's office," recalled Joseph Russin, referring to Kennedy aides Arthur Schlesinger Jr., class of 1938, and McGeorge Bundy, who served as the dean of the faculty at Harvard before Kennedy tapped him as national security adviser.

Kennedy's presidency—the rise and fall of Camelot—was the backdrop for some of the most extraordinary events in the lives of Huston Smith, Andrew Weil, Richard Alpert, and Timothy Leary. Kennedy was elected in the fall of 1960, the same season that Andrew Weil and the Harvard class of 1964 moved to Cambridge and began their undergraduate studies. On the very day Kennedy defeated Richard Milhous Nixon and was elected president, November 8, 1960, Aldous Huxley and his psychedelic connection, Humphrey Osmond, met with Leary and decided to work with him on the Harvard Psilocybin Project.

Russin was the president and editor in chief of the *Harvard Crimson* at the height of the Kennedy presidency. He would graduate, get hired by *Newsweek*, and head out to Berkeley in 1964 to cover the Free Speech Movement—the campus protests at the University of California that kicked off a decade of unrest at schools across the nation. Just a year earlier, at Harvard, such a thing was inconceivable to Russin. "Going out to Berkeley was a big cultural change for me. It was a totally different place. Berkeley was action and organizing. Gestures mattered more than well-reasoned arguments, which was the way we did things at Harvard."

Russin's last big story at the *Crimson* would involve two psychology professors named Alpert and Leary, but a staff writer named Andy Weil proposed the investigation and did most of the digging. To Russin, it seemed like a strange story for Weil to be covering. Until then, Weil had mostly done arts coverage for the paper—theater reviews and things like that. He had also worked as an editorial writer on the opinion page. Weil is best remembered not for his *Crimson* journalism but as an overweight, cigar-chomping practical jokester. At the time, a ribald rivalry raged between the *Crimson* staff and the kids over at the *Harvard Lampoon*. The famous satirical magazine has a statue of an ibis on top of its building. "Andy stole the bird," Russin said. "Then we'd take pictures of it in various locations and send the photos over to taunt the *Lampoon*."

Weil was *not* kidding around when it came to his opinions about Leary and Alpert's research project. "Andy came to me when I was president of the *Crimson* and told me that he thought we really ought to look into what Leary and Alpert were doing," Russin recalled. "They were giving LSD to students who were undergraduates, including some who were psychologically on the fence, some of whom were going nuts. There was a guy on *Crimson* staff who had been hospitalized for a mental condition after getting LSD from the Leary and Alpert crowd. Andy thought there was more of this, and either way, they were not following the deal they made

with the university, which was not to give the drugs to undergraduates."

Andrew Weil deserves most of the credit—or blame—for being
the guy who brought down Leary and Alpert. But he was not the
first *Crimson* reporter to break the story about all the controversy
surrounding their drug research. One year before Weil got onto
the case, in the spring of 1962, another *Crimson* editor, Robert E.
Smith, broke the first story on the dispute raging within the Center
for Research in Personality over Leary and Alpert's research methods. Smith's roommate, Graham Stellwagon, an undergraduate
studying under Alpert, tipped him off.

Graham was one of the heavier drinkers in their dorm. In one
drinking session of soon-to-graduate seniors, he told Smith about a
strange scene that was developing around Leary and Alpert.

"There's a clique there. You might even call it a cult," he told
Smith. "You should check it out. There's a real in crowd. Some are
in and some are out. I'm out, that's for sure."

"I don't get it, Graham," Smith replied. "What's the story?"

"How the hell do I know? I'm not in the in crowd. But there
is something going on. Leary and Alpert are taking some kind of
pills with a bunch of students."

Smith got interested and started thinking about how he could
get more inside information. He'd been covering the university administration, sports, and state politics—not intrigue within academic departments.

Then Graham gave him the lead he needed to break the story
wide open.

"There's this prof over there, Herbert Kelman, who doesn't like
what's going on," Stellwagon said. "Actually, they're having this big
showdown meeting about Leary and Alpert's research. I think it's
next week sometime. I can get you the details. It's at this old mansion over on Divinity Avenue. Just slip into the meeting. It's just

supposed to be for people in the department, but they never said it was off limits to outsiders. Chances are nobody will even notice you."

Smith was worried that he might be seen as an interloper, but he decided to give it a shot. Throughout his senior year, as the top editor at the *Crimson,* he had been on shaky ground with the university president and several faculty members. He was nonconfrontational by nature. If anyone at the meeting asked him who he was, Smith wouldn't lie. He expected that he might be asked to leave.

David McClelland had convened the March 14, 1962, gripe session in an effort to calm things down over in the Department of Social Relations, the university division that included the Center for Personality Research. There were two camps in the department— those taking the drugs, and those who were not. Opposing Leary and Alpert in the department were Herb Kelman and another professor named Brendan Maher.

Leary couldn't stand Maher. "I'm sick of these old lab rats, these dour experimentalists," he said. "If they had their way, we'd still be teaching students the way they were back in the Middle Ages." Leary thought Kelman was just jealous because all the bright students were gravitating toward him and Alpert. "What does he expect?" Leary said. "Who wants to spend two years filling out his lame questionnaires?"

At first glance, the intradepartmental dispute looked to be one of those petty personality clashes that often break out among faculty members working in the ivory tower. But there was a bit more to this controversy. Kelman believed that Leary and Alpert had gone way beyond the confines of scientific research. To him, it looked like they were starting a drug cult, promoting an ideology of spiritual enlightenment through modern chemistry. McClelland called the showdown meeting after Kelman reported that some students in the department had complained that they felt pressured into taking hallucinogenic drugs.

"You've got to do something," Kelman told McClelland. "These drugs are dangerous. One student was almost ready to kill himself after one of their sessions."

David McClelland was surprised when he walked into the room to convene the meeting. The place was packed. *Where did all these people come from?* he thought.

The turnout made it easy for Smith to slip into the session. There were far more undergraduates at the meeting than anyone expected. So no one seemed to care that Smith was sitting in their midst, furiously scribbling in his reporter's notebook.

McClelland started out the session by saying that he wanted to clear up a few misconceptions about Leary and Alpert's drug research. "I've gotten reports that some graduate students feel as if they are obligated to participate in this research," McClelland said. "Well, that is not the case. This is not part of the clinical program. If anything, participating in this project could harm you in your future career."

Kelman, a lecturer in social psychology, was anxiously waiting on deck. "I wish I could treat this as scholarly disagreement," he said, "but this work violates the values of the academic community. The whole program has an anti-intellectual atmosphere. Its emphasis is on pure experience, not on verbalizing findings. It is an attempt to reject most of what the psychologist tries to do. I'm also sorry to say that Dr. Leary and Dr. Alpert have taken a very nonchalant attitude toward these experiments—especially considering the effects these drugs might have on the subjects. I am not at all impressed by the way they are administering this project. What most concerns me, and others who have come to me, is how the hallucinogenic and mental effects of these drugs have been used to form a kind of 'insider' sect within the department. Those who choose not to participate are labeled as 'squares.' I just don't think that kind of thing should be encouraged in this department."

Richard Alpert responded to Kelman's critique. "With all due respect, Dr. Kelman, I must differ with your contention that our work violates the values of the academy and the university. Harvard has long been considered a fearless leader in providing a climate of encouragement for exploration and discovery. I see our research as right in the tradition of William James. These drugs we are studying are the most powerful consciousness-altering substances known to man. They certainly deserve our most serious and creative attention. In the tradition of William James, we are working toward the development of new models to conceptualize these profound mind-manifesting experiences. There is nothing to fear here. We have adequate safeguards, and no students or subjects have been coerced into participating in our research. Our procedures have already been looked at and approved by the Food and Drug Administration, the University Health Services, and the Sandoz labs, the synthesizer of the psilocybin we have used in these experiments. We are studying these substances to find ways they may be safely used to further man's growth and education. What could be more important for the future work in the psychological and sociological studies? How is this *not* in line with our task here at Harvard? Let me also say that the personal attacks that have been leveled against our research not only violate our academic freedom; they border on slander."

Smith couldn't scribble notes fast enough. It was a tense meeting, and it went on for nearly two hours. Smith checked his watch. The deadline at the *Crimson* for making the morning edition was 10 P.M., but that could be pushed to 1 A.M. for major stories for the front page. Smith was determined to get the story in the next day's edition, but he was nervous about what he was about to publish. As the top executive at the *Crimson,* he had regular meetings with Nathan Pusey, the president of Harvard. Pusey had also made himself acting dean of the faculty, replacing none other than McGeorge Bundy, who held the dean's post until he left the university to go work in the Kennedy White House. Pusey had tried to censor stories before, but he wouldn't get a chance this time. Smith was the reporter, but Smith was also in charge. He had been the top editor on the daily student paper since the previous January. He had already reserved space on the front page in the next morning's paper, even though he couldn't really explain earlier in the day what the story was going to be about.

At one point in the meeting, Leary declared that psilocybin could be used in nursing homes and hospices to ease the dying experience of the elderly. In fact, the drug could actually make the dying process ecstatic. Smith didn't have much time to think about framing his story, so he thought fast. On the one hand, the whole discussion seemed like a civilized debate, on a high level, over academic freedom and new frontiers of discovery. It seemed like the "clique" aspects were secondary. Still, the lives of young people—or at least their well-being at college—were at stake. The young journalist wasn't sure who was right—Alpert or Kelman—but he knew the debate was an important one.

Everyone who was at the meeting was shocked to see their internal dispute splashed across the pages of the morning paper. The story was published in the March 15, 1962, edition of the *Crimson,* under the headline, "Psychologists Disagree on Psilocybin Research." Smith reported: "Members of the Center for Research in Personality clashed yesterday in a dramatic meeting over the right of two colleagues to continue studies on the effects of psilocybin, a consciousness-expanding drug, on graduate student subjects. Opponents of the studies claimed that the project was run nonchalantly and irresponsibly and that alleged permanent injury to participants had been ignored or underestimated."

It didn't take long for other newspapers to pick up on the story. The very next day, the *Boston Herald,* a Hearst tabloid, ran an article under a more sensational headline: "Hallucination Drug Fought at Harvard—350 Students Take Pills." Actually, the story reported that 350 "subjects" had taken the drug. Many of them were not students, but the psychedelic cat was out of the university bag.

Smith published one follow-up story on the dispute, reporting on May 28 that Alpert and Leary had agreed to have a faculty committee "advise and oversee" future research on psilocybin. Medical doctors with the University Health Services had already taken possession of Leary and Alpert's psilocybin pills. Alpert was quoted in the story as saying that he and Leary hoped to "establish guidelines to make us and the rest of the University comfortable about the project."

Smith graduated in June. Most of the campus community disappeared for the summer, and it looked as if the controversy surrounding Alpert and Leary had been put to rest.

But this story, as they say in the newspaper business, had legs. The controversy surrounding the two rebel psychologists was far from over. Other events were unfolding. Alpert had gotten involved with Ronnie Winston, the undergraduate and former roommate of Andrew Weil. Classes resumed in the fall, and a new crop of reporters started trying out at the *Crimson.*

Like Russin, Bruce Paisner, the new managing editor that fall, was surprised when Andy Weil approached him about following up on the story that Robert Smith had done the previous year. Paisner was befuddled on a couple of levels. First of all, Weil was not a news reporter. He'd always seemed more interested in theater and other artsy stuff. On the other hand, Weil had written a couple of science stories, a subject most of the liberal-arts students working at the paper had trouble covering. Nevertheless, Paisner was skeptical about the story Weil now wanted to write. He talked it over at an editorial meeting at the *Crimson* office.

"Something's funny here," he said. "Is this real? Why has Andy suddenly shown up here so excited about this story?"

Paisner, who would go on to a career as a top executive with the Hearst Corporation in New York, had other reasons to be confused. He had never heard of "psychedelics" or some drug called "psilocybin." He *had* heard of marijuana, which was seen at the time as the dangerous drug everyone was supposed to be worrying about. So he sat down with Weil to get more details about the controversy.

"So what is this drug we're talking about here, Andy?"

"It's a different sort of drug," Weil replied. "It distorts the mind. It produces hallucinations."

"Really?" Paisner said. "Talk about your New Frontier. OK. There may be something there. Why don't you check into it some more and get back to us?"

Neither Paisner nor Russin, who replaced Robert Smith as the new president of the *Crimson,* knew that Weil himself had run a series of psychedelic drug tests just around the corner from the newspaper office during his freshman year, over at Claverly Hall. And Paisner didn't have a clue that Weil was moonlighting as a spy for the Harvard administration, helping President Pusey get the goods on Richard Alpert. He also didn't know that the undergraduate whom Weil was pressuring to testify against Alpert was Ronnie Winston—his old friend from Claverly.

"All of us who were active at the newspaper saw the administration at Harvard in a largely adversarial light," Paisner would later say. "We regarded our job as shining bright lights in dark corners, wherever they might be. I would not have sanctioned going out undercover as a *Crimson* reporter and then turning over information to the administration."

Russin, who went on to work as a manager at the *Los Angeles Times* and several West Coast television stations, *did* know that Weil was helping the university administration gather evidence against Alpert. "We did turn over a lot of stuff to the university after the article ran. In retrospect, we probably shouldn't have done that. But at the time, it seemed like the right thing to do. My reason was I had become convinced that these guys shouldn't be there and that we should help the university out on it. But we had a lot of trouble getting people to talk. I had the impression that something cultish was going on at the house out there in Newton. So I didn't have qualms about turning some of our research over to the university. But if this had all happened ten years later, I probably wouldn't have done it."

Weil had various motives for going after Richard Alpert. "For whatever reason," he says, "I got into this role as investigative reporter. The university really wanted to get rid of Alpert. They were looking for something to use against him, and they didn't have anything. At the same time, the Massachusetts criminal-justice people got wind of the stories and they were looking into it. They wanted to subpoena our files. So, under pressure from this criminal investigation, we decided we'd just turn our information over to the university. They called all the people we mentioned in our reports and everyone denied everything except this one undergraduate [Ronnie Winston] who said Alpert had given him this drug on this occasion. Alpert had given him psychedelics after promising not to give them to undergraduates. That's what they used to fire him."

Alpert says he was not all that surprised that Weil was the guy who brought them down. They never trusted him. "Andrew Weil wanted very much to take the drugs. Tim and I had a discussion that this was a guy at the *Crimson* who probably just wanted to get a story. So we said no."

What enraged both Ronnie Winston and Richard Alpert were the tactics Andrew Weil used to get his former friend to incriminate Professor Alpert.

"Andrew kept simmering about our relationship," Alpert said. "He went to Harry Winston, Ronnie's father, and he said, 'Your son is getting drugs from a faculty member. If your son will admit to that charge, we'll cut out your son's name. We won't use it in the article.'"

So, under pressure from his father, Andrew Weil, and the *Crimson,* Winston reported to the dean's office, where he was asked:

"Did you take drugs from Dr. Alpert?"

"Yes, sir, I did," Ronnie confessed. "And it was the most educational experience I've had at Harvard."

Years later, Weil would confirm Winston and Alpert's account of what happened. He would explain that the *Crimson* had to get someone to tell the truth about what was going on with Leary and Alpert. "Everyone else we had information on said they would deny everything. Ronnie was the only person who might confirm what we had. So we went to his parents. We talked to Harry and told him that this was probably going to appear in the press, and there was a chance that Ronnie would be named in all this. Harry got Ronnie to go in and talk to the dean, so we said we could keep his name out of it."

Weil's attack on Leary and Alpert did not stop at Harvard and the college newspaper. He went on to get national exposure by writing another article, "The Strange Case of the Harvard Drug Scandal," and getting it published in *Look* magazine in November 1963. In that piece, Weil reveals all kinds of inside information about the drug scene at Harvard and the details of Alpert's undergraduate liaisons. But he never reveals that *he* was a big part of that undergraduate drug scene. Weil writes in *Look* that students were getting mescaline from the supply houses that did few background checks on their customers, never mentioning that he was one of those customers. Weil also does not reveal that he was a friend of the undergraduate who testified against Alpert, and that he pressured his friend into doing so.

"One Harvard junior told a friend that Alpert had persuaded him to take psilocybin in a 'self exploratory' session at Alpert's apartment," Weil wrote in *Look*. "There were stories of students and others using hallucinogens for seductions, both heterosexual and homosexual."

About a decade later, Weil published his first book, *The Natural Mind: A New Way of Looking at Drugs and the Higher Consciousness.* He begins the book by revisiting that remark in *Look* about Alpert and the "stories of seduction, both heterosexual and homosexual," and offered an apology. "There were stories of students and others doing many other less titillating things with hallucinogens, but I picked that one for its journalistic value, and *Look* printed it for the same reason," Weil writes. "When I gave up the point of view of a journalist, I came to see that it was one of the most distorted ways of interpreting observations about drugs and I resolved not to make use of it again."

That apology was an olive branch to Leary and Alpert, but Weil did not come clean about his role in the whole affair. He blames "journalism." He does not mention that he violated journalistic ethics by failing to reveal his role in the Harvard drug scandal and by working as an undercover agent for one of the institutions he was reporting on for the student newspaper. A reporter's intent is an important factor in judging a journalist's ethics, not to mention an important consideration in libel law. In this case, there was a motive and at least the possibility that Weil got onto this story with "malicious intent."

Nearly half a century after Weil brought down Leary and Alpert, Winston and others involved in the affair were still mad about the whole series of events. "I hope Andrew Weil is ashamed about what he did," said Paul Lee, sitting in his backyard in Santa Cruz, California, in the spring of 2008. "He is the top guy on my list to punch out if I ever meet him. He was a spy for the administration. He went around interviewing people, including me, then reported it to the administration. I told him things candidly and in confidence and he betrayed me. He submitted my interview to the authorities. That was dirty pool. He was just out to get fame by doing in Leary and Alpert."

Andrew Weil was only eighteen years old when he first walked into the offices of the Center for Research in Personality and volunteered to be a research subject in Leary's psychedelic study. Weil would go on to graduate from Harvard Medical School and become a best-selling author. His career would take off when he emerged in the 1970s as an expert, sympathetic witness for the burgeoning drug culture. He replaced Leary and Alpert as the most trusted advice doctor for connoisseurs of recreational drugs. Decades later, Weil's books on holistic health and natural living would put him on the cover of *Time* magazine and on such television programs as *Oprah* and *Larry King Live.*

Only in retrospect does it become clear that Weil's career began with his betrayal of Ronnie Winston. He scored points with the university in his crusade to gather incriminating evidence against Leary and Alpert. His university career began, and Leary and Alpert's ended, on the night of May 27, 1963, when Weil and his

*Crimson* editor knocked on the front door of Alpert's house and presented the professor with a copy of the exposé they were planning to run in the next day's newspaper.

Accompanying the news story was a devastating, unsigned editorial written by Weil and Russin. It accused Leary and Alpert of being "propagandists" prone to "making the kind of pronouncement about their work that one associates with quacks." Alpert was singled out for "behavior that is spreading infection throughout the academic community.

"The shoddiness of their work as scientists is the result less of incompetence than of a conscious rejection of scientific ways of looking at things. Leary and Alpert fancy themselves prophets of a psychic revolution designed to free Western man from the limitations of consciousness, as we know it. They are contemptuous of all organized systems of action—of what they call the 'roles' and 'games' of society. They prefer mystical ecstasy to the fulfillment available through work, politics, religion, and creative art. Yet like true revolutionaries they will play these games to further their own ends."

Weil's journalistic scoop and editorial assault got the attention of newspapers across the nation. It put Leary and Alpert on the national media map as the leaders of a counterculture rebellion that would help define the 1960s. Weil's investigation focused the attack on Leary and Alpert. At the same time, the two Harvard researchers were probably destined to leave the restrictive confines of the university, with or without the investigative zeal of Andy Weil. They needed a bigger stage.

Seeker
Newton, Massachusetts
Spring 1963

Richard Alpert, Timothy Leary, and the other folks living in the big white house on Kenwood Avenue—the same home Weil visited with a copy of his exposé—were more than just roommates. Strong

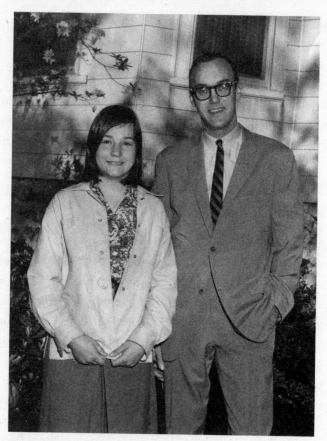

*Susan Leary, the daughter of Timothy Leary, stands next to Richard Alpert outside the house on Kenwood Avenue on May 28, 1963, the day after Andrew Weil's exposé in the* Harvard Crimson *got Leary and Alpert kicked out of Harvard. (Photo by Robert Backoff,* Boston Globe.)

bonds tend to form among people who share psychedelic drugs. Taken under the right conditions, psilocybin mushrooms, mescaline, Ecstasy, LSD, and other mind-altering drugs break down the protective wall that the ego builds around the self. This powerful experience can be both terrifying and transformative. It can drive an unstable person over the edge, and it can spark extraordinary levels of interpersonal communion.

All of these things were happening to the students, faculty, and other research subjects who took psychedelic drugs under the supervision of Timothy Leary and Richard Alpert. So it didn't take long for their research project to morph into an extended family, spiritual community, religious cult, and, finally, social movement. Many of Leary and Alpert's students wanted to live together, and love together, so Alpert purchased another large home in Newton, just around the corner from Leary's rented house on Homer Street, at 23 Kenwood Avenue.

They were both living there when Weil's story broke in the *Crimson,* but Leary was already away setting up the next stage of the crusade. Alpert was fired for giving drugs to an undergraduate. Leary was officially relieved of teaching duties for "leaving Cambridge and his classes without permission." Where was he? Leary had already removed himself to the Hotel Catalina, a funky seaside resort in Zihuatanejo, Mexico. There, his psychedelic storm troopers would continue their explorations under the mantle of a new organization called the International Federation for Internal Freedom.

Meanwhile, back in Boston, Alpert was left holding down the fort on Kenwood Avenue. Leary left his two young children, Jack and Susan, in Alpert's care—establishing a pattern that would continue for the next several years. Leary's kids would have a front-row seat for the psychedelic revolution that Alpert and Leary were about to lead. Filling out the Kenwood Avenue commune were an assortment of Harvard students and other hangers-on, including Barbara and Foster Dunlap, a young couple with a sixteen-month-old child.

It had been nearly three years since Leary first tasted magic mushrooms at his summer villa south of the border, so Mexico seemed like a good place to go and seek shelter from the storm. Leary and Alpert had been kicked out of Harvard. Now their Newton commune's neighbors were on the warpath. This was a single-family neighborhood, not the kind of place that welcomed

a tribe of troublemakers who played loud music and were coming
and going at all hours of the night. Alpert had purchased the house
himself and moved in during the fall of 1962. It didn't take long
for the good people of Newton to see that something strange was
going on inside the house. They filed a complaint with the city that
the occupants of 23 Kenwood Avenue were living in flagrant viola-
tion of the town's zoning ordinance. Richard solicited the represen-
tation of his father, George Alpert, the well-known Boston lawyer,
businessman, and Jewish philanthropist, to represent the commune
members. Yes, Alpert argued, there were a total of twelve people
living in the home—eight adults and four children—but they
considered themselves "a single family." George Alpert appeared
before the Newton board of zoning appeals on February 26, 1963,
just three months before his son got kicked out of Harvard. Alpert
stood before the board in his three-piece suit, thumbs in the watch
pockets, looking like Clarence Darrow. He was a well-known
lawyer, not to mention president of the New Haven Railroad. "This
is the Family of Man," he proclaimed, "but a family nonetheless."
In this family, the renowned lawyer explained, the five men did
the shopping and washed the dishes, while the three women did
the cooking and housework. Money was contributed to a common
fund, Alpert said, according to the means of the individual. This
seemed like a very radical idea at the time—at least to the *Boston
Herald,* which proclaimed: "BIG 'FAMILY' STIRS PROTEST:
Men Do the Dishes in Newton 'Commune.'"

Richard Alpert and the Family of Man won that battle. They
appealed the Newton eviction order and won in court. But the
powers that be at Harvard and the city fathers of Newton were
right in one way. Alpert and Leary and their growing family were
living too large for Harvard to contain them. This Family of Man
was too universal to fit into a single-family home on the leafy streets
of Newton.

———————

Residents of the Kenwood commune shared more than the house-work. One account of life in the house reports that "Alpert was in love" with Foster Dunlap, who, like Winston, was an undergradu-ate at Harvard. According to Alpert, it was not that simple. Yes, he said, there was a strong and loving bond between the people living in the Kenwood Avenue house. Taking psychedelic drugs together on a regular basis will do that. Casual acquaintances become soul mates. The connection may have a sexual component, or it may not. It almost doesn't matter. Years later, Alpert tried to describe the relationship.

"Barbara and Foster were lovers. You see, in cases like this I was not an actively sexual partner. But there was an intimacy that came with the experience. It was the same kind of thing with Ronnie. We were psychedelic lovers."

It was the kind of connection that Grace Slick, the female vo-calist with the Jefferson Airplane, would sing the praises of a few years later in the David Crosby free-love anthem, "Triad." *Sister lovers. Water brothers. And in time, maybe others . . . I don't really see; why can't we go on as three.*

The unorthodox scene inside the Kenwood Avenue home, and in the larger cult that was starting to form around Leary and Alpert, was an early warning sign of a counterculture movement that would soon sweep across the nation. It would be a social up-heaval fueled in no small part by two powerful pharmaceuticals: LSD; and that other pill, the birth-control pill. Many forces would forge the changes that were about to rock America in the 1960s, yet few would be as important as drugs and demographics. The baby boomers, whose story would keep sociologists and other trend spotters busy well into the new millennium, were just starting to come of age. Sexual roles, living arrangements, and family struc-tures were about to undergo rapid, revolutionary changes. But the changes wrought by psychedelics are not just matters of the mind. They can transform the way we live and love.

Ralph Metzner was living in the Kenwood Avenue commune with a woman who would become his wife. But in some deeper way, he felt married to the larger group. Tripping together opened up a kind of communication that blended into a spiritual communion. Everyone in the house felt a deep connection. Sometimes that would be expressed sexually. Other times it wouldn't, but they were all in love. Metzner, his future wife, and a few other members of the household went out to Cape Cod one weekend to trip together. They camped out on the beach, built a bonfire, and took psilocybin. They felt so bonded after the session that no one wanted to leave. "Why don't we all get married?" Metzner said the next morning. "Let's start with the two of you and the two of us and go from there."

Another member of the Kenwood Avenue family, Peggy Hitchcock, would have a major role in the next chapter of the psychedelic saga. Hitchcock, along with her brothers, William and Tom, were heirs to the banking and oil fortune amassed by Andrew Mellon, the Pittsburgh industrialist, and Mellon's nephew, William Larimer Mellon, the founder of Gulf Oil. Peggy and her brothers would become Alpert and Leary's primary patrons after the two renegade professors were kicked out of Harvard. Peggy met Tim in early 1962 at a New York salon frequented by actors, artists, and jazz musicians. They became close that summer, when Hitchcock first flew down to Mexico with Leary and Alpert to establish their south-of-the-border retreat in Zihuatanejo.

Peggy was instantly attracted to Leary. He was absolutely charming, so bright and funny and charismatic. *So* charismatic. Hitchcock was swept off her feet by Leary's charm, and by his psychedelic vision. The young heiress was an instant convert. Peggy longed to share this feeling, this profound experience they were having, with all of mankind. They could change the world.

Peggy Hitchcock would follow the psychedelic family from Kenwood Avenue to Mexico and finally to a vast estate in upstate New York that her brother William bought and turned over to Leary. Tim and Peggy would be on-and-off lovers over the next few years. To her, the people who gathered around Leary and Alpert did seem like a family, but Hitchcock kept looking back at the other family—what was left of Leary's original family follow-ing his wife's suicide back in Berkeley in 1955. That family tragedy had yet to play itself out, but Peggy saw what was there, and it was not good. She was in love with Tim, and was thinking about marrying him, but she just couldn't accept the way he related to his children. It was a red flag. He was dismissive of the kids. He spent very little time with them. He didn't have time for that. He was on his own voyage of self-discovery.

Taking care of the kids was Alpert's job. Hitchcock saw how Richard cared for the kids, how much he loved them. He was much more of a nurturing type than Leary. Peggy had romantic feelings for Richard, too, but Alpert's preference for male love kept that relationship in check.

Kenwood Avenue became the new command center for the psychedelic revolution after Leary and company got kicked out of the house over on Homer Street. The professor who'd rented it to Tim returned from his sabbatical and found the place trashed. There were those burn marks on the floor around the fireplaces in the living room, dining room, and study. There were busted wall lamps and big scuff marks on the white ceiling of the third floor from the days when Leary's son, Jack, would come home with his friends from their football matches and continue the game indoors. Jack liked to play catch on the third floor with Lafcadio Orlovsky, who lived in the house for a time with his brother, Peter Orlovsky, Allen Ginsberg's lover. William Burroughs, the writer and heroin addict, was holed up in one of the rooms for a while.

Leary and Alpert didn't have a landlord or returning professor to worry about at the Kenwood Avenue house. Major renovations were possible there, so Leary decided to construct a special cham-ber for his ongoing experiments with psilocybin, LSD, and DMT (dimethyltryptamine), the latest drug to be added to the communal medicine cabinet. DMT is a powerful, short-lasting hallucinogen that was administered intravenously. Psychedelic sessions were held in the new trip chamber Leary built on Kenwood Avenue. The residents sealed off and wallpapered over the only door leading into one room. Leary then climbed in through the window with a chainsaw and cut a small hole in the floor. The window was covered over and wallpapered, so the only way to get into the chamber was to climb up on a ladder from the cellar. There were nothing but mattresses and cushions on the floor. A dim light illuminated a bronze Buddha statue donated by Peggy Hitchcock. Completing this prototype of the hippie crash pad were lots of Indian bedspreads and a seemingly unlimited supply of incense. The idea was to create a transcendental community whose members would fully experience life and go beyond routine ego trips and social games. Two of the leading graduate students involved in the Harvard Psilocybin Project, George Litwin and Gunther Weil, moved into a sister community with other devotees on nearby Grey Cliffe Road.

There seemed to be a magical connection between the sister homes and the rest of the early psychedelic family living in the neighborhoods around Harvard. One night, Huston Smith was tripping in the special chamber Leary had built over at the Kenwood Avenue house when a burning candle ignited one of the Indian bedspreads. Suddenly, Huston found himself stoned on acid and sitting before a wall of flame. He was able to put the fire out and make it out the escape hatch and down the ladder, but it was a close call.

That same night, Huston's wife went to bed in the couple's home in Belmont, Massachusetts, miles away from the Kenwood Avenue commune. At one o'clock in the morning, Kendra Smith woke up with a start. She smelled smoke—a strong smell of smoke. She got up and ran down to the basement to check the furnace. Everything was fine. The smell was so strong that she almost called the fire department, but she felt too embarrassed to report a fire when she couldn't even find the smoke. So she went back to bed.

Huston told her about the Kenwood Avenue fire only the next morning, when he returned home from his trip. To Kendra, the events that night seemed like a psychic experience—a feeling that often accompanies the ingestion of a psychedelic drug.

Leary and Alpert's transcendental community in the Boston suburbs was a harbinger of the hippie communes that would pop up across the country in the late 1960s. But it also harked back to an earlier social experiment conducted not far from Newton, in the Roxbury section of Boston.

One hundred and twenty years before Leary and Alpert established their three homes in Newton, a transcendentalist and former Unitarian minister named George Ripley founded Brook Farm, a utopian community organized in the 1840s—the same decade in which Henry David Thoreau set up camp at Walden Pond. Leary would soon come to see his life as a continuation of the work of Thoreau, Emerson, and Margaret Fuller, the American writer and protofeminist who participated in the Brook Farm experiment.

Leary and Alpert liked to compare their ouster from Harvard with the earlier banishment of Ralph Waldo Emerson, who wore out his welcome with a famous 1838 address to the graduating class at Harvard Divinity School. In that speech, Emerson condemned the odious errors of historical Christianity, calling its depiction of the Son of God a "noxious exaggeration." True religion, Emerson proclaimed, would allow "every man to expand to the full circle of the universe." Twenty years after he was kicked out of Harvard, Leary would cite the transcendentalists as the inspiration behind his call that every man "turn on, tune in, drop out."

"They, too, were saying turn on, tune in, go within. Become self-reliant. Before Emerson came back to Harvard in 1838, he was in Europe hanging out with notorious druggies like Coleridge and Wordsworth," Leary said at a 1983 Harvard reunion. "They were expanding their minds with hashish and opium and reading the Bhagavad Gita. Then he came back here and gave that famous speech where he said, 'Don't look for God in the temples. Look within.' Find God within yourself. Drop out. Become self-reliant. Do your own thing."

Leary was notorious for his overstatements, grandiose thinking, and inflated sense of his own place in the universe. After all, this was a guy who had enough chutzpah to stand in front of a New York City theater marquee that proclaimed, "Dr. Timothy Leary—Reincarnation of Jesus Christ." But at the same time, the iconoclastic Leary truly was following in the footsteps of Ralph Waldo Emerson. So it's not surprising that Harvard University—founded by Puritans and nurtured as an exclave for the Protestant elite—was not quite ready for Richard Alpert and Timothy Leary. Neither were their neighbors on Homer Street, Kenwood Avenue, or Grey Cliffe Road. This early chapter in the psychedelic sixties was coming to an end, and the band of gypsies would have to find somewhere else to go.

# CHAPTER FIVE

# Trouble in Paradise

Trickster
Zihuatanejo, Mexico
Summer 1963

Leary and Alpert had been kicked out of Harvard, but that wouldn't end the research, nor would it stop the party. It was summertime, and time for the second season of Tim and Richard's psychedelic summer camp. Their tropical encampment had been inaugurated in the summer of 1962, when they packed Peggy Hitchcock into Alpert's Cessna and flew down to this sleepy beach town north of Acapulco, checking into the Hotel Catalina. This year, hardly pausing after their expulsion from Harvard, Leary and Alpert started spreading the news about a second summer session down on the Mexican Riviera. But this year was different. There would be no Harvard classes for these two professors to go back to in the fall. No more professional prestige. Those days were gone. It was time to start anew, and what better place to do it than in the land of the magic mushroom.

For Ralph Metzner, the German grad student who was quickly becoming a full partner in Leary and Alpert's crusade, Mexico was a refreshing change from all the psychodrama back at Harvard. They tripped amid the exuberant lushness of the Mexican jungle, within earshot of the ceaseless rhythm of the surf. They reveled in extravagantly beautiful sunsets, silent lightning storms over the Pacific, and the sweet aroma of exotic flowers. It was a mythic setting, especially when experienced through psychedelic lenses. Women were transformed into sea nymphs or mermaids, while the men became Aztec warriors and jungle shamans.

It was a little piece of paradise, and that was exactly the idea. Leary no longer saw Mexico as an exotic place to escape for his summer vacation. Life among the three dozen pilgrims gathered at the Hotel Catalina was to be patterned after the utopian vision described in Huxley's final novel, *Island,* which had just been published the previous year. It's the story of a cynical reporter who gets shipwrecked on a mysterious Pacific island where the residents live in cosmic harmony with each other and the cosmos. The book was the counterpoint to *Brave New World,* Huxley's futuristic best seller in which the populace was controlled by an authoritarian regime using a mind-numbing drug called Soma. On Huxley's mythic island, the natives take *moksha*-medicine to tune into the wonders of the world with "pure receptivity."

LSD replaced psilocybin as the focus of Alpert and Leary's research in Zihuatanejo. In one session on a hotel balcony, Metzner took a moderate dose. With Leary as his guide, Ralph waited anxiously for the LSD to take effect. Tim was starting to see that people on acid could get beyond the limits of the obsessive mind by focusing on sensory awareness. In one of Metzner's sessions, Leary simply lit a candle. *What wonder!* He'd open a cool bottle of beer and hand it to Ralph—not to drink, but simply to touch. *So cool! So calming!* Metzner looked into Leary's eyes and saw the face of some godlike being. *How amazing! Such radiant light!* Then he'd suddenly see that half of Leary's face was terrifyingly ugly. *Not just ugly. My God, he's demonic! Is this Satan? Is this heaven, or hell?*

Leary saw the fear in Metzner's face and calmly reassured his eager protégé. The teacher was sounding less like a professor, more like a guru: "Remember, both the fear and the light come from within you. Pretty soon you'll be able to see divinity in the whole face, or in this candle, or this cigarette, or the whole day."

Ralph Metzner calmed down. His identity and his awareness seemed to be spread throughout the room and even beyond, into the forest outside the hotel. When somebody came into his room, it was as if they were walking into his soul. They were accepted like thoughts entering his head. They would walk around in his head, and he'd examine their relationship with extreme equanimity. All these people were just parts of himself. Seeing that was so powerful, so liberating, so psychologically healing.

Friends, academics, students, and other explorers of higher consciousness gathered at the Hotel Catalina, where you could check out anytime you liked, but you could never leave. For Peggy Hitchcock, it wasn't just some beach party. Sure, it was loads of fun. There were times of joy and excitement. But there was a purpose to it all, a higher discipline. They were not just getting high. They were transforming themselves into another kind of being.

For Leary, it was a glimpse of utopia, a glimmer of something that would not last. At first, they felt like they were living out Huxley's vision in *Island*. But before long, the scene began to feel more like *Brave New World*. That peaceful, easy feeling soon gave way to creeping paranoia.

It started out fine. There were the usual psychiatrists and students signing up for sessions, plus a Hasidic rabbi and a businessman trying to kick a booze habit. They took acid once a week, then spent the rest of the time discussing their experience, strumming guitars, playing chess, and listening to talks on the history of mysticism. But Leary and Alpert's ouster from Harvard had gotten international media attention, and the trickle of guests soon turned into a flood. All that publicity inspired a wave of protohippies to wash up onto their shores. They arrived broke and unkempt, begging for food, shelter, and cosmic illumination.

According to Leary, the real trouble began when a mysterious woman named Mary Pinchot Meyer failed to appear for a scheduled visit to Zihuatanejo. Meyer was a Washington, D.C., socialite, the former wife of a CIA agent named Cord Meyer, and an intimate friend to President Kennedy. One of the more sensational stories in Leary's 1983 autobiography, *Flashbacks*, is his claim that he supplied Meyer with LSD and that she used Leary's acid to turn Kennedy on in the White House.

In the early summer of 1963, Leary writes, he was in Zihuatanejo when he received a cryptic note from Meyer. "I won't be joining you," she wrote. "Too much publicity. Your summer camp is in serious jeopardy." Leary says Meyer warned him that the federal government was cracking down on his psychedelic crusade. "It's the publicity. I told you they'd let you do anything you want as long as you kept it quiet," she purportedly told Leary. "But they're not going to let CBS film you drugging people on a lovely Mexican beach. You could destroy both capitalism and socialism in one month with that sort of thing."

Leary goes on to write that Meyer called him following the Kennedy assassination. "He was learning too much," she said over the phone. "They'll cover everything up. I'm scared. I'm afraid."

Mary Pinchot Meyer was murdered in a Washington, D.C., park on October 12, 1964, eleven months after the Kennedy assassination.

Regardless of whether one chooses to believe Leary's tale, there was enough factual evidence to keep conspiracy theorists busy for decades. Leary *did* have an early encounter in Berkeley in the 1950s with Cord Meyer, who *would* go on to become a CIA division chief and marry Mary Pinchot. The CIA *did* conduct its own LSD research at Harvard a decade before Leary discovered psychedelic drugs. It appears that Mary Pinchot Meyer *did* have an LSD session with Leary, and that she *did* have an affair with John F. Kennedy. And, for whatever reason, the Mexican authorities *did* kick Leary and the crew out of the Hotel Catalina and out of the country in the summer of 1963.*

---

*The CIA had already funded its own psychological research at Harvard. One of its most infamous subjects was an undergraduate named Theodore Kaczynski, aka the Unabomber. In his book *Harvard and the Unabomber: The Education of an American Terrorist,* Alston Chase documents how Kaczynski's participation in CIA-funded psychological stress tests in the 1950s contributed to his mental breakdown. Those experiments were run by the influential Harvard psycholo-

## Seeker
## Millbrook, New York
## Fall 1963

Not only had Alpert and Leary been kicked out of Harvard. Now they had been booted out of Mexico. Later that summer, their efforts to set up shop on Antigua and Dominica abruptly ended with their eviction from those Caribbean islands. They would soon laugh at how they'd been kicked out of one college and three countries in three months. Years later, Leary and Alpert would get their federal intelligence files under the Freedom of Information Act. It turns out that the CIA had tracked them all the way down to Dominica, where the agency reported that the professors planned to open "an alleged Happiness Hotel."

"We should have hired the CIA as our press agent," Alpert quipped.

Their summer exodus across Mexico and the Caribbean turned out to be a blessing in disguise. Timothy Leary and Richard Alpert would soon find their promised land on a twenty-five-hundred-acre estate in Dutchess County, New York. They had found Millbrook, and they were about to turn it into the Disneyland of the psychedelic sixties.

Millbrook's crown jewel was a sixty-four-room Gothic mansion built around the turn of the century by William Dietrich, a manufacturer of carbide lamps. Located about eighty miles north of New York City, the white, four-story building is an architectural jumble of towers and turrets surrounded by a broad veranda. The interior is busy with hand-carved woodwork and faded tapestries. It has ten bathrooms. There are orchards, pine forests, a waterfall, horse stables, and various other buildings, including a three-story

---

gist Harry Murray, who during World War II worked for the Office of Strategic Services, the precursor of the CIA. Late in his Harvard career, Murray was one of the few members of the Harvard faculty who volunteered to participate in Leary's psilocybin experiments.

gatehouse and a chalet containing a bowling alley. Leary described the place as "Bavarian baroque."

It was provided as a refuge to Leary, Alpert, and their growing entourage by Peggy Hitchcock and her two brothers, William and Tommy—their patrons and trust-fund millionaires. Profits from Gulf Oil—one source of the family fortune—were now fueling the psychedelic crusade. At Peggy's suggestion, Alpert turned William Hitchcock onto acid and into a key supporter of their cause. Who needs Harvard when Mellon's millions are backing you up? William and Tommy would come up from Manhattan on the weekends to unwind in a four-bedroom cottage about a mile away from the main mansion, which was eerily empty when Peggy and Alpert first explored its labyrinth of rooms one night using candlesticks for illumination.

Over the next three years, Millbrook would provide the backdrop for Leary and Alpert's psychedelic drug research. During this period, legal access to LSD would get more and more difficult, inspiring Leary to sponsor a series of seminars in which other methods of consciousness expansion were employed, such as meditation, dance, breathing exercises, and sensory deprivation. Guests would pay sixty dollars to sit and meditate in the many empty rooms of the main house.

Down in sunny Mexico, the utopian society Huxley envisioned in *Island* provided a guidebook for guests at the Happiness Hotel. Up in woodsy Millbrook, a more fitting model was found in Hermann Hesse's final novel, *The Glass Bead Game*. This futuristic story unfolds in Castalia, a remote region set aside for the intellectual elite to achieve advanced personal development in philosophy, music, and the arts. Leary and Alpert established a new organization at Millbrook, the Castalia Foundation, to continue the consciousness-raising campaign they began with the International Federation for Internal Freedom. Appropriately enough, Castalia was also the name of a sacred spring near Delphi, whose waters were used to inspire the muses of ancient Greece.

Hesse was a major influence on Leary, as was the Armenian

mystic G. I. Gurdjieff. One of the exercises performed at Millbrook was based on the Gurdjieffian strategy of using shock tactics and puzzling games to awaken initiates out of their normal way of thinking and experiencing the world. One trick at Millbrook was to serve the paying guests green eggs and black milk for breakfast. Another was to require that everyone immediately stop what they were doing or thinking whenever Ralph Metzner would strike a bell that would echo throughout the main house.

Paul Lee was visiting Millbrook one weekend with Huston Smith, who had packed Lee and his entire family into their van and headed up to check out the scene. At one point during the weekend, Lee was sitting in the house chatting away with Huston about how he was never really sure why he got into the study of religion. "Maybe it was all because my grandmother and grandfather got divorced, and broke my mother's heart," Lee said to Huston. "I started flirting around about going into the Lutheran ministry, probably for the sake of my mother. I'd been studying philosophy at St. Olaf College in Northfield, Minnesota, and for some reason decided to go to Luther Theological Seminary in—"

Then, out of the blue, Metzner rang the bell. "GONG!"

At first, Lee was pissed off at the rude interruption of his story.

"Jesus, man! What are you doing?" he asked Metzner. "We were just having a conversation!"

Lee then remembered that this was all part of some psychospiritual exercise. As instructed, he stopped and began reflecting on his nonverbal experience of the moment. That in itself was something new to the verbose professor. Lee would later recall that weekend as an important turning point in his life. And it happened simply because Metzner rang a bell and Lee started exercising the nonverbal side of his brain.


There was another experience that weekend that was not so profound. It was an unpleasant encounter that Lee had with Van Wolf, a New York entrepreneur and talent agent who had first introduced

Leary to Peggy Hitchcock. On this weekend, Leary and Alpert had run out of LSD, which was a big disappointment to Wolf. It turned out, however, that Lee *did* have some LSD. Leary had previously given him a couple of hits, and Lee had brought it up to Millbrook. Wolf was sniffing around for some LSD, and Lee made the mistake of mentioning that he had some. Wolf really wanted it and got very agitated when Lee wouldn't give it to him.

William Hitchcock had just bought a new station wagon. Wolf got ahold of the keys and said, "Who wants to take a ride? Let's take a ride!" So a small gang piled into the station wagon, including the brother of Nena von Schlebrügge. Nena was a tall, blond fashion model, the daughter of a Swedish baron. She would later become Leary's third wife in a marriage that would last less than a year. Nena would then marry Buddhist scholar Robert Thurman and give birth to a daughter who would grow up to become actress Uma Thurman.

Van Wolf tore down the road and into the backcountry of the vast Millbrook estate, stopping first at the cottage of jazz trumpeter Maynard Ferguson, who lived at the Millbrook estate with his wife, Flo. He emerged from the cottage with some extremely potent pot, which everyone in the car proceeded to smoke while Wolf drove around the property, getting totally ripped.

It was a Sunday night, and there was a religious program on the radio. A choir sang the hymn "Our Father" as Wolf kept driving faster and faster, swerving from one side of the road to the other. Lee wasn't sure if Wolf was engaged in one of Metzner's psycho-spiritual exercises or if he was just being a stoned jerk. He was swerving so much on the dirt road that he finally banged the car into a tree.

"Does anyone want to go over any of that again?" Wolf asked.

"No, Van, that's enough." Lee replied.

Wolf responded by backing up, throwing the car into drive, and ramming into the tree again. Then he backed up farther to give himself even more room to accelerate into the same tree a third time.

By now, the whole front of the car was bashed in.

"That's enough, Van!" Lee yelled.

Wolf backed up and ran into the tree again.

Lee felt like he was being held hostage by some terrorist. *"Don't hit the tree, Van!"* Finally, they headed back to the house. One whole side of the car was smashed, and the tailpipe was dragging along on the ground. When they got back, Lee headed up to his room to get away from the madman behind the wheel.

Wolf was determined. He burst into Lee's room.

*"I want your stuff and I want it now!"*

"No way, man," Lee said. "Get the hell out of here!"

Wolf left the room, but Lee lay in bed all night worrying that the guy was going to come back, kill him, and steal his acid.

Fulltime Millbrook residents normally faced no such shortages of LSD, especially the leaders of the pack. Leary and Alpert took a lot of drugs at Millbrook, but the idea—at least at first—was not just to get high. One of the effects Leary and Alpert were studying was LSD's ability to "imprint" new ideas and new behavior on the user—not just during the trip itself, but on a long-term basis. This was also one of the reasons the CIA was studying the drug.

Most learning is done through a long process of repetition, but what if LSD could be used to instantly "imprint" new behavior on an individual? This could be of great benefit to society, curing people of alcoholism or helping to reduce the recidivism rate among criminals. It could also be used as a sinister means of social control. One could imprint upon a hapless victim the idea that he should assassinate a foreign leader, a story line played out in the 1962 film *The Manchurian Candidate.* Both the CIA and the Castalia Foundation soon discovered, however, that it was not so easy to control the psychological insights or the psychotic terror one experiences with psychedelic drugs. Users may be blasted into a higher state of consciousness that completely transcends their previous mental constructs and social conditioning. But it is very difficult to turn that insight into long-term behavioral change.

In one of his more extreme psychedelic experiments, Alpert locked himself in the bowling alley at Millbrook with five other test pilots. They took a huge dose of LSD (four hundred micrograms) every four hours for two weeks. The idea was to see if they could finally break through their mental conditioning and become a different kind of human being. They soon discovered that they quickly built up a tolerance for LSD. They could get only so high on repeated megadoses. The other finding from the bowling-alley experiment was even more discouraging. After two weeks of constantly dosing themselves, the test subjects came to thoroughly hate each other. It was the beginning of the end of the dream. Alpert was starting to see that LSD would not save the world.

Alpert's experiment in the Millbrook bowling alley occurred in 1965, when both Leary and Ralph Metzner were off on pilgrimages to India. Leary's journey was also a honeymoon with Nena, the Swedish model. As usual, Alpert was left behind to take care of Leary's kids. He was also left in charge of Nena's mother, brother, and the strange assortment of druggies, artists, psychologists, and other mystical explorers who came to Millbrook to find The Answer, or to at least get high.

Leary's return would mark the end of his five-year partnership with Richard Alpert.

Metzner had already left on his own journey to the Far East. He and Leary returned to Millbrook in the summer of 1965 and were shocked at what they found. In their view, Alpert had converted Millbrook from a community of scholars and scientists to a playground for rowdy omni-sexuals. The place had been taken over by street-tough New Yorkers using LSD for mischievous fun.

Metzner came home and was met at the front door by a strange man wearing clothes Ralph had left behind. He soon realized that Millbrook had split into two camps. There was the camp of Alpert and his friends. They were into mind fucking—using psychedelics to manipulate other peoples' minds. At staff meetings they'd say things like, "I'm telepathic and can tell you're lying." In Ralph's view, everything they had cultivated before—openness, sharing, companionship—had turned around into manipulation. One group just wanted to be high all the time. They didn't want to sweep the floor and do the dishes. Then there was another group of commune residents who, as Metzner saw it, were trying to keep some kind of order.

Adding fuel to the fire were Leary and Metzner's concerns about Alpert's sexual appetite. Metzner had come to see that Alpert had this tendency to idealize young men. "He'd fall in love with these guys," Metzner would later recall, "and he'd say, 'Oh. He's my guru now. Tim's not my guru anymore.'" Metzner wouldn't use the word *gurus* to describe the guys Alpert had brought into the scene. Words like *idiots* and *punks* were closer to the mark.

Alpert and Leary's partnership did not survive Tim's return to the chaotic scene at Millbrook. They had developed an almost telepathic relationship, but it was not to last. Leary was the first to acknowledge that Alpert had taken on a maternal, wifelike role with his kids. Tim had to concede that his own children were closer to Richard than they were to him. But it suddenly dawned on Leary that the children had been eyewitnesses to all the craziness on the New York estate.

Jack Leary was fifteen years old when his father returned from India. Part of the problem was that Tim was never comfortable with Richard's eclectic but mostly gay sexuality. He got this idea in his head that Alpert had been seducing his son. Jack insisted there was no seduction under way, but Tim wouldn't drop the matter. At one point, he accused his son of being gay.

"No, dad, I'm not gay," Jack replied. "And even if I was, there's nothing wrong with being gay."

Alpert reached the breaking point when Leary sat down with him and his children in Susan's bedroom in Millbrook and uttered the words "Uncle Dick is *evil*."

"Oh, come on, Dad," Jack Leary replied. "Uncle Dick may be a jerk, but he's not evil!"

Alpert turned to Leary. "If you really think I'm evil," he told his own mentor, "you must be psychotic."

Whether Alpert was evil or not, psychotic or sane, it was the bitter end of the Leary and Alpert show. Alpert had devoted five years of his life to Leary's vision. He'd sacrificed his coveted Harvard career. He'd given Tim and the psychedelic cause all his money. And here was his reward—being told he was "evil" in front of two children he had loved and nurtured while Leary was running off chasing women and promoting himself. He'd had enough. He'd baked the bread. He'd taken care of the children. He'd held the hands of all the women Leary seduced and left behind. And now he was being told that he had to leave Millbrook because he was "evil."

Alpert had gotten kicked out of Harvard, Mexico, Antigua, and Dominica. Now he was getting booted out of Millbrook. But he'd learned some important lessons. LSD was not going to save the world. Their grand experiment in new forms of communal living and loving-kindness had dissolved into rants of recrimination and a paranoid atmosphere of mutual distrust.

Now what?

Alpert loved playing the loyal lieutenant. He excelled at being the number-two man. In a few years, he would head off to India and find a new guru, but in the meantime, he was out on his own. There would be one more chapter in his life, and in the lives of the rest of the Harvard Psychedelic Club, before Richard Alpert made his storied journey to India and returned as Ram Dass. It was 1965. The whole world seemed to be heading out to San Francisco, with or without flowers in their hair. Richard Alpert decided to just go with the flow.

# CHAPTER SIX

# If You Come to San Francisco . . .

Trickster
San Francisco
January 1967

Timothy Leary was at the top of the bill for the great Gathering of the Tribes for a Human Be-In at the Polo Fields in Golden Gate Park, leading a line-up that included Richard Alpert, Allen Ginsberg, Jerry Rubin, Gary Snyder, the Grateful Dead, and "all of San Francisco's rock bands." It was here, dressed in white, with beads around his neck and a yellow flower tucked behind his ear, that Leary made his first public appearance in San Francisco and delivered the slogan that would follow him around for the rest of his life. Stoned on three hundred micrograms of LSD, Leary looked out from the stage, which was covered with oriental rugs, and into a crowd of twenty thousand furry freaks gathered under a brilliant winter sun. "Drop out of high school. Drop out of college," he said. "Drop out, junior executive. Drop out, senior executive. Tune in, turn on, and drop out!"

His messianic appearance at the counterculture classic capped an incredible thirteen months in the life of Leary. It began with his arrest at the Mexican border in December 1965 and his conviction four months later, and continued with him testifying before a U.S. Congress determined to stamp out the burgeoning LSD subculture. In June 1966, at an LSD conference in San Francisco, the event at which Huston Smith would sound his cautionary note on the direction of the psychedelic movement, Leary was as enthusiastic as ever. He predicted that within one generation the University of California at Berkeley would have a Department of Psychedelic Studies.

His advice that the youth of America "drop out" would prove to be the most controversial component of that counterculture trilogy, and it did little to bring about a "gathering of the tribes." Many people assume that the tribal references in the Human Be-In promotional material referred to the burgeoning interest in Native American spirituality among the baby boom generation. That's only half true. The gathering in Golden Gate Park was also a strategic move designed to bring together the "hippie" and "political" wings of the youth movement. The event was announced in the *San Francisco Oracle,* an underground newspaper that chronicled the midsixties psychedelic scene in San Francisco like no other journal of its time. It called for a coming together of "Berkeley political activists and the hip community and San Francisco's spiritual generation and contingents from the emerging revolutionary generation all over California." These were the tribes that were to ecstatically come together in a "union of love and activism previously separated by categorical dogma and label mongering."

Writing in the next issue of the *Oracle,* Stephen Levine described the actual scene at the Human Be-In. "Bare foot girls in priest's cloaks, madras saris, and corduroy. Teenage braves stripped to the waist in a hot winter sun. Folksingers charting mountain ranges in their imaginations. Shamans and motorcyclists, lovers and voyeurs, cowboys and Indians, cloud of gold-yellow incense geysers from the stage."

Levine had come to San Francisco from New York in 1964, stopping first in Mexico to kick a heroin habit he'd picked up back in Greenwich Village. He would later emerge as a fellow traveler with Richard Alpert and become a popular writer and meditation teacher in his own right. "Psychedelics were a godsend," he would later say. "They showed people another level in themselves that they thought was just a fairy tale."

Leary's self-appointed role as the messiah of that psychedelic godsend did not go unquestioned. Many felt Tim had gone overboard
and was bringing on the heat. Some felt Leary's main motivation
was his own fame and fortune. Peace-movement activists called for
demonstrations against Leary and his apolitical stand. Writing in
*Ramparts* magazine, journalist Warren Hinkle mocked Leary as
the "pretender to the hippie throne." At one public appearance, a
woman pelted Leary with eggs, yelling, "You ruined my son with
your devil drugs!" Even Allen Ginsberg, who worked with Leary
in the early days of the Harvard campaign and shared the stage
with him at the Human Be-In, was starting to question Tim's slo-
ganeering. He put Leary on the spot during a debate held on the
Sausalito houseboat of Alan Watts one month after the Human
Be-In. "Everybody in Berkeley," Ginsberg said, "is all bugged because they say this drop-out thing really doesn't mean anything,
that what you're gonna cultivate is a lot of freaked-out hippies goof-
ing around and throwing bottles through windows when they flip
out on LSD."

But Leary could not be stopped. He was determined to secure
his position as the high priest of the LSD movement. He knew
he needed the news media to spread the psychedelic gospel, and
journalists knew they needed Leary to figure out whatever it was
that was going on in the early years of the counterculture. Leary's
concern for public relations was on display the night following the
Human Be-In in San Francisco, when he ran out to get an early
edition of the *San Francisco Chronicle.* He rushed the newspaper
over to an apartment in the Haight-Ashbury area where Ginsberg,
Gary Snyder, and others were in the midst of a postcelebration
party.

Leary handed the newspaper to Ginsberg, who read the story,
headlined "HIPPIES RUN WILD," and let out a moan. "That's
ridiculous," Ginsberg complained. "Like, it was an aesthetically
very good scene. They should have sent an art critic."

Ginsberg picked up the phone and called the newspaper to register his complaint with the night editor at the *Chronicle*.

"What is this nonsense about hippies running wild?" Ginsberg asked the befuddled editor. "Your story has the kind of inaccuracy of tone and language that's *poisoning* the community. Is *that* what you want to do?"

"We sent our hippiest reporter," the night editor replied.

"I don't know what kind of hippies you've got over there at *your* place," Ginsberg said, chuckling. "Besides, what is this 'hippie' business? What does 'hippie' mean, anyway? These kids aren't hippies—they're seekers. Today was a serious religious occasion."

Ginsberg promised to go over to the newspaper first thing Monday morning and talk to the reporter about doing a more accurate follow-up story. The editor said that would be fine. They'd see the famous poet at the *Chronicle* offices on Monday.

"Well, peace," Ginsberg said, hanging up the phone.

Ginsberg, still dressed all in white, was sitting on a mattress in the meditation room in the apartment of Michael Bowen, one of the Be-In organizers. The mattress and the wall behind him were covered with Indian bedspreads. Sitting next to him was Gary Snyder, who had beads hanging over his turtleneck sweater. Most of the people at the party were still in their Be-In costumes, except for Leary, who had taken off his loose white garments and changed into a sports jacket and trousers. That wardrobe change made him look more professorial when the television news crew showed up dragging klieg lights and cables into Bowen's apartment.

The cameraman turned away from Leary and held a light meter up to Ginsberg's face. Here was a guy with a bushy black beard, love beads, and white robes. Better visuals for a TV news segment on the hippies.

The poet groaned at the TV crew. "Man," he said, looking at Bowen, "it's bad enough that you have a *telephone* in your meditation room."

Ginsberg lightened up when the TV reporter offered his take on the day's festivities. "I don't know why," the television guy said, "but this whole day strikes me as absolutely sane and right and beautiful. You guys must have put something in my tea."

"What's so insane about a little peace and harmony?" Ginsberg replied. "Thousands of people came to the park today, just so they could relate to each other—as dharma beings. All sorts of people—poets, children, even Hell's Angels. People are lonely. It's strange to be in a body."

Gary Snyder nodded. "People are groovy," he said.

Ginsberg looked into the television camera. "It was very Eden-like today," he said. "Kind of like Blake's vision of Eden. Music. Babies. People just sort of floating around having a good time and everybody happy and smiling and touching and turning each other on and a lot of groovy chicks all dressed up in their best clothes and—"

"But will it *last*?" the reporter asked.

"How do I know?" Ginsberg said. "And who cares?"

Leary's media strategy for the promotion of LSD was devised with an assist from Marshall McLuhan, the Canadian communications theorist and the influential author of *The Medium Is the Message*. Over lunch at the Plaza Hotel in New York, McLuhan critiqued Leary's dreary appearance before two Senate subcommittees. Keep your message positive, McLuhan advised, and keep smiling. "Wave reassuringly. Radiate courage. Never complain or appear angry," he told Tim. "You must be known for your smile." Leary listened to McLuhan, and became a major American media personality. Pictures of him appeared in countless newspapers during the mid-1960s and into the 1970s, and the most striking thing about that photo record is how Timothy always has this radiant smile spread across his face. He may be getting arrested. He may have just been hit with a thirty-year prison sentence. But he's always smiling.

Leary's major media coup of 1966 was a lengthy interview published in the September issue of *Playboy,* in the same edition that featured a photo spread about the topless nightclub scene that had erupted in the North Beach entertainment district of San Fran-cisco. The *Playboy* interviewer had come to Millbrook to meet with Leary during the spring, and he found him "reciting Hindu morn-ing prayers with a group of guests in the kitchen of the 64-room mansion." Leary led his guest up to the third-floor library, through an open window and onto a mattress placed on the tin roof of a second-story bay window. They made themselves comfortable on the double-width mattress, listening to the song of a chickadee in a nearby tree before beginning their conversation. Leary opened his shirt to the warm sun, wiggled the toes of his bare feet, and awaited the first question.

PLAYBOY: How many times have you used LSD, Dr. Leary?

LEARY: Up to this moment, I've had 311 psychedelic sessions. . . .

PLAYBOY: We've heard about sessions in which couples make love for hours on end, to the point of exhaustion, but never seem to reach exhaustion. Is that true?

LEARY: Inevitably. . . .

PLAYBOY: How often have you made love under the influence of LSD?

LEARY: Every time I've taken it. In fact, that is what the LSD ex-perience is all about. Merging, yielding, flowing, union, com-munion. It's all lovemaking. You make love with candlelight, with sound waves from a record player, with a bowl of fruit on the table, with the trees. You're in pulsating harmony with all the energy around you.

PLAYBOY: Including that of a woman?

LEARY: The three inevitable goals of the LSD session are to dis-cover and make love with God, to discover and make love with yourself, and to discover and make love with a woman. . . .

PLAYBOY: According to some reports, LSD can trigger the acting out of latent homosexual impulses in ostensibly heterosexual men and women. Is there any truth to that, in your opinion?

LEARY: On the contrary, the fact is that LSD is a specific cure for homosexuality. It's well known that most sexual perversions are the result not of biological binds but of freaky, dislocating childhood experiences of one kind or another. Consequently, it's not surprising that we've had many cases of long-term homosexuals who, under LSD, discover that they are not only genitally but genetically male, that they are basically attracted to females. The most famous and public of such cases is that of Allen Ginsberg who has openly stated that the first time he turned on to women was during an LSD session several years ago. But this is only one of many such cases. . . .

PLAYBOY: We've heard that some women who ordinarily have difficulty achieving orgasm find themselves capable of multiple orgasms under LSD. Is that true?

LEARY: In a carefully prepared, loving LSD session, a woman will inevitably have several hundred orgasms. . . .

PLAYBOY: Have you allowed or encouraged [your two children] to use marijuana and LSD?

LEARY: Yes, I have no objection to them expanding their consciousness through the use of sacramental substances in accord with their spiritual growth and well being. . . .

PLAYBOY: How will this psychedelic regime enrich human life?

LEARY: It will enable each person to realize that he is not a game-playing robot put on this planet to be given a Social Security number and to be spun on the assembly line of school, college, career, insurance, funeral, goodbye. . . . Man is going to have to explore the infinity of inner space, to discover the terror and adventure and ecstasy that lie within us all."

Those were just a few of the many provocative statements Leary made in the lengthy interview, which shocked even the most sympathetic scientists studying the effects of LSD. It would be cited by psychedelic research proponents as one of the many Leary actions that helped bring a total federal ban on LSD research. Did Timothy Leary really mean what he said in the *Playboy* interview? What was he really up to? Was he just playing the trickster? Late in his life, Leary looked back on everything he'd said over the years and compared his level of truthfulness to the batting average of major-league baseball players. "About a third of what I've said is just flat-out bullshit," he told a friend. "About a third of what I've said is just dead wrong. But a third of what I've said have been home runs. So I'm batting .333, which puts me in the Hall of Fame."

By the summer of 1966, Leary felt like he had nothing to lose. He was already facing a thirty-year prison sentence that, at the age of forty-five, was basically a life sentence. He told *Playboy*, "Since there is hardly anything the middle-aged, middle-class author-ity can do to me—and since the secret is out anyway among the young—I am free at this moment to say what we've never said before: that sexual ecstasy is the basic reason for the LSD boom."

But there *was* more that America could and would do to Timothy Leary.

Seeker
San Francisco, California
Summer 1966

It was way past midnight on one of those magic nights at the Fillmore. The Jefferson Airplane was jamming with the Grate-ful Dead, about halfway into an extended version of the Wilson Pickett tune "Gonna Wait 'til the Midnight Hour," when Joan Baez, who was in the audience, jumped onstage and started sing-ing along with them. *I'm gonna wait 'til the midnight hour. That's when my love comes tumblin' down.* Richard Alpert was danc-ing wildly on the ballroom floor, staring lovingly into the eyes of Caroline Winter, a young hippie girl he'd met earlier that eve-ning. They were spinning around together, stoned out of their minds, as hundreds of revelers formed a human chain and danced around them. Colors swirled. Minds did, too. "Look at those faces shine," Alpert screamed over the music, flashing a wide grin at his dance partner. "They're angels! Look! Look at the wings. They're angels!"

Richard Alpert settled into the swinging San Francisco scene the year before Leary finally made his messianic appearance at the Human Be-In. On the night Alpert met Caroline Winter, these concerts, celebrations, dance parties at the Fillmore Auditorium, an old ballroom on Geary Street, had been happening for about six months. They were the brainchild of a young music promoter named Bill Graham, and they were something new. "Acid Rock" was born amid the early flowering of the hippie scene in little pockets around the San Francisco Bay, but it took root in this ballroom and in the nearby Haight-Ashbury neighborhood in San Francisco. The old music scene in San Francisco had been a few jazz clubs and poetry-reading venues and coffee houses frequented by the Beats. This was different. The drugs were different. Red wine was so yesterday. Orange sunshine was today, here and now. It fueled these Dionysian rites at the Fillmore, starting with the first concert on December 10, 1965—a benefit in support of the San Francisco Mime Troupe that featured the Jefferson Airplane, the Great Society, and the John Handy Quintet.

On this night, in July 1966, the bands that came to personify the San Francisco sound—the Jefferson Airplane and the Grateful Dead—were sharing the bill. For Caroline Winter, who would soon become Richard Alpert's first and only steady girlfriend, it was the beginning of one of those soon-to-be-infamous, long, strange trips.

Caroline was born in England in the middle of World War II. She grew up in the aftermath of those devastating years, when British society seemed exhausted, gloomy, and class ridden. Sure, the Beatles and the Rolling Stones livened things up during her college years, but Caroline was ready for something completely different. After college, she was accepted into graduate school in England, but on a whim she decided to head out to California instead. She arrived in Berkeley in September 1965.

She landed in town with very little money and took the first job she could find, in a local real-estate office. Her life changed one afternoon when some guys from a band called the Warlocks came by looking to rent a place where they could rehearse. Caroline fell in with the band, which was about to change its name. Inspired, like Leary and Alpert, by an ancient Buddhist tome, the Tibetan Book of the Dead, the band started calling itself the Grateful Dead. They soon outgrew their Berkeley studio and moved across the bay into an old Victorian at 710 Ashbury Street, where the Dead quickly became the house band for the psychedelic subculture that took root in the Haight.

On this summer night, Caroline arrived early at the Fillmore. She entered the auditorium on Geary Street, walking up a staircase to a little ticket booth, turned left, then up some more stairs to the second floor. Outside the ballroom, the entry hall was lined with glowing psychedelic posters advertising the coming attractions. Lenny Bruce had appeared the previous month, sharing the bill with the Mothers of Invention. In the coming week, Beat poet Allen Ginsberg would share the stage with Sopwith Camel. Caroline turned away from the posters and headed into the ballroom, where she was intercepted by Owsley Stanley.

That would be Augustus Owsley Stanley III, the underground chemist who'd gotten his start with the Grateful Dead. Owsley, as he was called, was the son of a government attorney and grandson of a U.S. senator from Kentucky. After a stint in the U.S. Air Force, he met Melissa Cargill, a UC Berkeley chemistry major who helped him produce his first batch of pure, powerful LSD. Owsley's acid became the central sacrament for the tribe gathering around the Dead. Operating out of a warehouse in Point Richmond, a town on the edge of the San Francisco Bay, they churned out nearly four million hits of acid during the mid-1960s.

"Open your mouth and shut your eyes and I will give you a big surprise," Owsley told Caroline, placing a tab of LSD into her mouth. "Come on. Let's go meet a friend of mine."

Owsley's friend was Richard Alpert, who'd moved out to San Francisco after his falling-out with Timothy Leary and the rest of the old tribe back at Millbrook. Leary would soon follow Alpert out to the West Coast, but the infamous Harvard duo were merely the best-known members of a huge westward exodus. A tidal wave of East Coast refugees came to the San Francisco Bay area between 1965 and 1968. The region hadn't seen anything quite like this since the days of the Gold Rush, back in 1849. Both events involved wild, outlaw migrations that attracted thrill seekers and people with nothing left to lose. More than a few of the midsixties migrants carried a little book in their backpacks titled *The Psychedelic Experience: A Manual Based on the Tibetan Book of the Dead,* written by Timothy Leary, Ralph Metzner, and Richard Alpert. The book, published in 1964, offered detailed flight instructions for initiation into the cult of LSD.

Alpert arrived in San Francisco and went straight to the Haight, just as the hippie revolution was taking form in this blue-collar neighborhood of dilapidated Victorians and struggling shops. Rents were cheaper than over in North Beach, where the edgy artists, Beat poets, and assorted hangers-on were losing their monopoly on hip. In Berkeley, on the other side of San Francisco Bay, the revolution was political and had a harder edge. It was mellow in the Haight. Golden Gate Park was just a few blocks away. Alpert offered his impressions in an article published in the *Oracle.*

"The Haight Ashbury is, as far as I can see, the purest reflection of what is happening in consciousness, at the leading edge in the society. There is very little that I have seen in New York, Chicago, Los Angeles, that is giving me the hit that this place is because it has a softness that is absolutely exquisite," Alpert wrote. "We are human beings who are making a statement about how we are going to live our lives, gently and lovingly."

On the night he met Caroline Winter, Alpert was at the Fillmore with Allen Ginsberg, who never seemed far from the sixties action. He had been there that night at the start of the Harvard Psilocybin Project. One night, stoned on the mushroom pills, Ginsberg tried to call John F. Kennedy from Leary's house and inform the new president that world peace was at hand. That was the same night the gay poet tore off his clothes and threatened to run naked through the streets of Boston—a stoned messiah with a message of love. The beat icon was back at the Homer Street house a few months later, when Alpert had his first psychedelic trip on the snowiest night of the year. And here he was five years later in San Francisco, hanging out at the Fillmore. On this night, however, Alpert and Ginsberg were looking for something other than a rock concert. Alpert's old pal from Millbrook, jazz trumpeter Maynard Ferguson, was performing over at the Playboy Club, so they decided to bring along Caroline Winter, who was just taking off on her very first LSD trip.

Caroline was sitting between Alpert, who was driving, and Ginsberg, riding shotgun. She was getting more and more stoned as they drove up and down the city's precipitous hillsides. She grabbed hold of her escorts' hands when everything started looking like it was upside down. Caroline was starting to freak out on this roller-coaster ride through the streets of San Francisco.

"This is too weird!"

"Don't worry, baby," Ginsberg said. "We are with you all the way."

Caroline was blown away by the entire experience that night, and soon fell in love with Richard Alpert. Over the last decade, Alpert had had more lovers and sex partners than he could remember. Most of them were men, some of them were women, but Caroline was one of the few real loves of his life. For Caroline, however, the relationship with an infamous, older, bisexual man was intense and confusing. Meeting someone as strong and charismatic as Richard Alpert was overwhelming enough. But it was all happening in a supercharged, psychedelic state of mind. Later, as her relationship with Alpert was deepening, Caroline got the news that her father had died back in England from a heart attack. Suddenly, she felt desolate and bereft, but Richard was there to help her through the grief.

They became a couple, and the relationship got serious enough that Alpert decided to have Caroline meet his parents back in Newton. They drove all the way across the country in October 1966 in Richard's antique Buick. Alpert's parents were polite, but

Caroline could tell they did not approve. They were glad to see that Richard had finally found *someone,* but couldn't he do better than that? Caroline was more than a decade younger than Richard. She wasn't Jewish. And to top it all off, she wore miniskirts. Mrs. Alpert did not approve of miniskirts. At the time, Alpert's mother was battling cancer and had a greatly enlarged spleen. Caroline got the sense that the woman was not long for this world—that she wanted to spend time with her son and not with some stray girl he'd dragged in behind him.

Caroline and Richard became closer after Mrs. Alpert's death. Both of them had lost a parent, and their shared experience deepened the bond. They rented an apartment in Manhattan for a few months, and even went up to Millbrook to see if Leary and Alpert could reconcile their estranged relationship. Tim and Richard tried to rekindle their friendship, tried to make it seem like the good old days, but Caroline could tell there was still a lot of tension between the two men. Leary presented a cheerful facade, but Caroline could see the tension behind the mask.

Not surprisingly, the Millbrook gossip centered on Alpert's return. Not only was he back at the grand New York estate; he had shown up with this little hippie *girlfriend.* Caroline could see that many of Richard's old friends were puzzled by her appearance and envious of the fact that she was so close to Richard. *What's so special about her? Oh, he'll get over her once some young stud comes along.* Caroline felt like she was on trial. She could see that their relationship was getting too complicated. At the time, Richard was attracted to both men and women. He and Caroline had agreed to have an open relationship. Caroline went along with the plan, but she was never really that comfortable sharing her love with any Tom, Dick, or Harry.

When Richard and Caroline showed up, Millbrook was in its final chaotic year. The place was so crowded that people were practically living on top of each other. Leary was struggling with mounting legal bills stemming from his December 1965 arrest in Laredo, Texas, when police found three ounces of marijuana hidden in the panties of his eighteen-year-old daughter, Susan. Four months later, a Texas jury saddled Leary with a thirty-year prison term. He was out on appeal when, just a month after that, in the wee hours of a Sunday morning, a squad of sheriff's deputies raided the Millbrook mansion.

There had been a party the night before—dinner around low tables and cushions in the oak-paneled dining room. Bob Dylan, the Beatles, and Ali Akbar blasted from big stereo speakers. Leary and the woman in line to become his fourth wife, Rosemary Woodruff, passed around a pipe of DMT. Guests splashed blobs of colored paint on the mansion walls. Chromatic patterns undulated. Men with longish hair tended to a roaring fire while beautiful women danced about with yogic grace.

Outside in the bushes, an assistant district attorney peered into the windows with a pair of binoculars, fascinated with the psychedelic light show illuminating the house. Movies were shown of cascading waterfalls, kids jumping on trampolines in slow motion, men jumping out of airplanes, and other scenes designed to heighten the psychedelic experience. The D.A. in the bushes was none other than G. Gordon Liddy, a former FBI agent who had taken to using his first initial and middle name in imitation of his hero, J. Edgar Hoover. At first, Liddy thought the guests were watching pornographic movies. Then he realized there were no naked women in the films. But something very weird *was* going on in there. Sometime after midnight, Liddy and four Dutchess County sheriff's deputies bounded up the stairs and into Leary's third-floor bedroom. Leary and three other guests were arrested after the squad found a small stash of marijuana in one of the bedrooms. The charges were eventually thrown out of court, but the publicity was a boon to Liddy's law-enforcement career. Later, in one of the most delicious ironies in the amazing life of Timothy Leary, Liddy would be convicted as one of the burglars in the Watergate scandal that brought down the presidency of Richard Nixon, the same man who had called Leary "the most dangerous man in America." Years later, to top it all off, Leary and Liddy would become friends and head out on the lecture circuit together—two ex-felons out to entertain an audience and sell some books.

Back in the sixties, however, Timothy Leary was at the top of G. Gordon Liddy's hit list. Dutchess County sheriffs raided Millbrook a second time in December 1967 and charged their landlord and partner in crime, William Hitchcock, with conspiracy to create a public nuisance. By then, Leary and his fourth wife, Rosemary Woodruff Leary, had decamped back to the Learys' old family home in Berkeley.

Leary and Alpert made frequent tours of the West Coast following their ouster from Harvard. In the fall of 1964, before their estrangement at Millbrook, they gave a series of lectures in San Francisco and Palo Alto where, according to a headline in the *San Francisco Chronicle,* they foresaw "A Day When LSD Is Like Aspirin." Actually, they never said that. Leary told the *Chronicle* reporter that he thought the intellectual elite of the next generation would usher in greater use of psychedelic drugs, and the general population of the generation after that would use them to attain higher states of consciousness. Both Leary and Alpert warned that "unprepared" users could suffer destructive, rather than constructive, consequences from these drugs.

Following his ouster from Millbrook, in late 1965, Alpert went on a solo lecture tour across the United States. At an appearance in a San Francisco nightclub, Alpert paced back and forth across the stage, tossing off witticisms like a psychedelic Mort Sahl. In his more sober moments, Alpert told the crowd that LSD can produce "a religious experience without any significant side effects on the human body," but, once again, he warned against "injudicious use of the drug." After the lecture he took questions from an audience that included aging beatniks, protohippies, and other seekers of truth. It was a stump speech, but one that almost never got delivered. Earlier that same day, Alpert had been tripping on a beach south of San Francisco and had lost track of time. He barely made it to the club, and when he arrived, he was still very stoned. He still had this very pleasant, oceanic feeling—so much so that when he looked out into the crowd, the audience members appeared as a wonderful school of colorful fish. Alpert was laughing a lot that evening, and the levity was infectious, but few people in the crowd realized that they were the butt of Alpert's private, hallucinogenic joke.

During the question-and-answer period, one very earnest looking fish/man stood up and addressed Alpert. It was a very technical question about endorphins, brain chemistry, and mental functioning. Alpert couldn't focus on the words, which started bubbling from the mouth of the fish/man like he was in some cartoon. At one point, Alpert noticed that the word bubbles had stopped coming out of the fish/man's mouth, and that he was standing there in the audience waiting for some kind of answer. There was a long pause. Alpert looked at the man, trying to get beyond all the words, but all he could see was a sweet and somewhat insecure fish standing there asking, "Do you love me?"

"Yes," Alpert answered. "I love you."

The crowd roared with laughter.

Next question.

At the time, Alpert was doing more than just lecturing about LSD. He was also transporting large quantities of the drug. He'd not yet come to the realization that LSD was too powerful to be played with in such a haphazard way. He was still telling himself that everything would be fine if his love went out with the acid. No one would be harmed. But Alpert was no longer personally directing psychedelic sessions whose love and safety he had control over. He certainly knew about bad trips. He had had some wicked ones himself. If he'd really stopped to think about it, he would have had to admit that he couldn't really control what happened after he passed along a shipment. Whom was he sending love out to? The distributor? People he'd never even meet?

At least he knew it was good acid. Alpert's supplier was Owsley Stanley. Owsley's LSD was unveiled at a series of "Acid Tests" staged in 1965 by the novelist Ken Kesey and his band of Merry Pranksters—events that lead up to the Trips Festival at San Francisco's Longshoreman's Hall in January 1966. Back at Harvard, Leary and Alpert had become infamous for their LSD research, but that campaign was cautious compared with the crusade waged by Kesey and the Pranksters. Hundreds, and then thousands, gathered in backyards, halls, and auditoriums around the Bay Area to drop acid, dance, and revel under psychedelic light shows that were fast becoming the stock-in-trade of such gatherings. Jerry Garcia, the lead guitarist with the Grateful Dead, was crowned "Captain Trips."

Something new was happening. These weren't just rock concerts. This was something else—more like a three-ring circus with a very thin line between the audience and the performers. One of them, eighteen-year-old Dan Millman, dove off a balcony, somersaulted under strobe lights, and rebounded off a concealed trampoline. Nearly everyone—on and off stage—were blasted out of their minds, so many of them weren't sure just what to make of the flashing figure flying through the air. (Years later, Millman would reappear as the bestselling author of *The Way of the Peaceful Warrior* and other New Age books.) Jerry Garcia would suddenly stop playing his guitar, staring down in amazement as strange sounds came out of speakers that weren't even hooked up. Before his eyes, a maze of cables and wires turned into a den of writhing snakes. Poetry and other pronouncements echoed from a series of speakers set up around the hall. Kesey and company hooked up tape recorders and tape loops with strange sound delays. It made you believe in magic, far-out beautiful magic.

Two watershed events in late 1966 and early 1967—the Love Pageant Rally and the Human Be-In—would follow the Trips

Festival and usher in the Summer of Love, when it seemed like the whole world came to San Francisco in search of peace, love, and another way of living. The Love Pageant Rally was held on October 6, 1966, the day LSD became illegal in California. More than two thousand people gathered in the Panhandle of Golden Gate Park, where they danced to the music of the Grateful Dead and Big Brother and the Holding Company, a local band who were featuring their new singer, a girl from Texas named Janis Joplin. The event was announced on the back page of the first edition of an underground newspaper called *P.O. Frisco*. The rally was the brainchild of a small band of writers and musicians who had observed a group of angry, sign-carrying hippies demonstrating outside of a San Francisco police station, protesting the recent bust of their commune. *Who needs this endless confrontation with authority? Let's try something else. Let's change the world with celebration, not confrontation. Let's party!*

*P.O. Frisco* was a mess of a newspaper, but it blossomed into the legendary *Oracle,* which featured idealistic explorations into the personal experience and social implications of mind expansion. The *Oracle* was right there at the dawning of the Age of Aquarius, when a new generation began its grand experiment with Native American shamanism, Eastern mysticism, communal living, utopian revolution, sexual liberation, and ecological awareness. The rainbow newspaper, filled with the swirling and twirling calligraphy of psychedelic art, left behind the source documents for an eclectic spirituality and social philosophy that still exerts a widespread—albeit subtle—influence on American society.

*P.O. Frisco* published its first edition on September 2, 1966. Its lead columnist was none other than Richard Alpert, who offered readers his personal reflections on the intricacies of LSD intoxication. Alpert was living in Berkeley at the time with Caroline Winter. He was still struggling with the "old Richard Alpert" and had not yet given birth to the man who would be Ram Dass. He started his column with a confession: "There are times when I am afraid to take LSD because I am so hung up, so paranoid, distrusting, guilt-ridden, caught up in the ego tentacles of power, greed and lust." He ended his article with a vision of a time when people "will be high more of the time whether using or NOT using psychedelic chemicals," when people are "so ecstatically involved in our Here and Now life that we hardly have time to take drugs anymore."

<br>

### Teacher
### Marin County, California
### Summer 1966

It was all too far-out for Huston Smith, the MIT philosophy professor and ordained Methodist minister. He'd come to San Francisco not with flowers in his hair, but to deliver a well-reasoned paper at a reputable academic conference. Huston's paper was titled "The Religious Significance of Artificially Induced Religious Experience." A preconference party was to be held at a mansion in Marin County, the woodsy suburb across the Golden Gate Bridge from San Francisco, where the hosts hoped to provide some appropriate music.

They hired the Grateful Dead.

About two hundred people gathered on the grounds and around the swimming pool of an estate nestled in the foothills of Mount Tamalpais. Paul Lee, one of the conference organizers, surveyed the scene and could hardly believe his eyes. There were all sorts of people in the crowd—grandfathers, grandmothers, parents, children, teenagers—and many of them were running around naked. Owsley, adorned in a powder blue jumpsuit, was in the house handing LSD out to anyone who wanted it. He spotted Lee, a large man, and walked up to him.

"Wow, man," Owsley said. "You have such a friendly and familiar face."

Lee, who does not suffer fools gladly, replied with something between a smile and a smirk. "Yeah, I know, man," he replied. "I was born that way."

Owsley tried to press some LSD into his new friend's hand, but Lee declined. He had to give a talk at the conference the next morning. Plus it was fun enough to just watch all the antics.

Everyone was standing around by the pool, coming onto the acid and waiting for the Grateful Dead to start playing. Then one of the hosts took the microphone and announced that the owners of an adjacent horse stable were about to call the police unless everyone moved their cars. They were blocking their driveway. The news was relayed to the partygoers, and there was a great groan from the crowd, like the moan of a tired elephant seal. Everyone was ready to just lay back, trip out, and tune into the Grateful Dead. Lee was terrified that the whole conference was going to fall apart right there. People would stumble out to their vehicles and, if they could get their keys into the ignition, start running into each other like a giant game of bumper cars. Then the police would come and throw them all in jail. Lee thought to himself, *This is the test. If everybody gets up and moves their cars without incident, we are going to get through this week.* Miraculously, everyone got up and moved their cars in an orderly fashion. They returned to the backyard, lay back, and the band played on.

The conference at the University of California offices in San Francisco went on as scheduled. But even before Huston delivered his paper, Lee could see that the distinguished philosophy professor was getting tired of the circus surrounding the early years of the psychedelic scene. What had been going on back east was bad enough. But this West Coast scene was out of control. These were bacchanalian rites, and they were going down on an unprecedented scale. It was downright Dionysian.

Huston no longer wanted to be associated with the social movement that was coalescing around Leary and Alpert and Ken Kesey and the Grateful Dead. Smith looked at all the sexual immorality inspired by Timothy Leary, Richard Alpert, and psychedelic religion and was reminded of what Friedrich Nietzsche said about Christ's disciples—how they "should look more redeemed." To

Huston's mind, steeped in the history of religious movements, Leary and Alpert's actions smacked of antinomianism, the Christian heresy that asserts that true believers are exempt from moral and civil law because they're already saved.

"Huston was a moralist," Paul Lee would later explain. "He thought this antinomian trend was something to criticize. We said, 'Oh, man. Come on, Huston. Lighten up. Just because you were born in China to Methodist missionaries.' But he thought that because he was identified with all this, he had to critically comment on it. He did, and he was right. A lot of lives were damaged. Huston sounded the sour note at the conference, but in retrospect, I think that was important. But at the time, everybody just sniffed at him."

Huston wasn't the only one amazed at the wildness of the psychedelic celebration in San Francisco. Paul Lee couldn't believe his own eyes. It was his first introduction to the whole West Coast scene. His first stop was the Psychedelic Bookstore on Haight Street. It all took him and most of the other East Coast scholars completely by surprise. They had no idea that all this had grown up in California. They were still buttoned-down Harvard guys. Here was a completely different style. There was none of that at Harvard. They had Joan Baez, who came and played her guitar in the apartment of Paul Tillich, the distinguished German theologian. They thought *that* was far-out. They were still into Pete Seeger and the Weavers. They didn't have a clue.

Lee had suggested the West Coast LSD conference to Richard Baker, who had also studied with Tillich at Harvard. Baker would go on to become Baker-Roshi, the abbot of the San Francisco Zen Center, but at the time he had a job putting on conferences for the University of California. The five-day program was supposed to be held at the Berkeley campus. In addition to the Huston Smith speech, it would feature a talk by Leary titled "The Molecular Revolution" and an address by Allen Ginsberg, "Consciousness Politics in the Void." At the last minute, university officials on the Berkeley campus saw Leary and Ginsberg on the schedule and started worrying about the revolutionary tone of the conference. Baker compromised and agreed to remove Ginsberg from the program, although the radical gay Jewish poet came anyway and hung out all week. Baker also agreed to move the program from the Berkeley campus to a less official venue in San Francisco.

Serving on the conference advisory committee with Paul Lee and Huston Smith were Richard Alpert, Frank Barron, and Dr. Sidney Cohen, who had emerged as a leading voice of caution warning that the psychedelic revolution was spinning out of control.

Cohen, Alpert, and *Life* magazine photographer Lawrence Schiller had just published a short, point/counterpoint book debating the wisdom of the psychedelic revolution and the prospects for its future. The book, simply titled *LSD,* was filled with photographs that Schiller took of young people stoned on acid. Alpert, who revealed in the text that he had ingested psychedelic chemicals 328 times over the last five years, made a series of predictions, some of which came to pass. He said LSD would spark new interest in Eastern thought, music, and art, "along with the increase in popularity of Eastern methods of expanding awareness such as yoga, diets, meditation, and karate." Alpert was less on the mark when he envisioned the creation of "Ecstasy Centers" where people could gather to *legally* explore psychedelic drugs.

Cohen predicted, accurately, that the next few years would see greater consumption and greater abuse of the drug. "The hedonistic cults take over, the dance gets wilder, anything goes, the music is louder, the strobe lights flash faster," Cohen wrote. "Let's not speak of the dangers."

By the time Huston flew to San Francisco to deliver his paper, the tide had already turned in the public debate over LSD. Media coverage had shifted, and a drug that once offered "instant nirvana" was now portrayed as a dire threat to the mental health of an entire generation. The truth was, of course, somewhere in between, but the middle road is rarely taken once *Time* magazine and congressional subcommittees get into the act. *Time* declared in March 1966 that the nation was in the midst of an LSD epidemic. "The disease is striking in beachside beatnik pads and in the dormitories of expensive prep schools," *Time* intoned. "It has grown into an alarming problem at UCLA and on the UC campus at Berkeley. And everywhere the diagnosis is the same: psychotic illness resulting from the unauthorized, non-medical use of the drug LSD-25."

This is not to deny that there were many real casualties from the psychedelic drug craze. Millions of young Americans were turning on, and hundreds of them were showing up in hospital emergency rooms, suffering from panic attacks and psychotic reactions. Others complained of LSD "flashbacks," the onslaught of hallucinations weeks or even months after taking the drug. In New York, the news media went into overdrive in the spring of 1966 when a Harvard graduate and medical-school dropout named Stephen Kessler stabbed his mother-in-law to death with a kitchen knife. According to media reports, the "LSD killer" told police he'd been "flying for three days on LSD." There were reports of freaked-out users jumping off of buildings or taking their lives in other ways under the influence of the drug. The most famous casualty would be Diane Linkletter, the daughter of television personality Art Linkletter, who jumped to her death from the kitchen window of her sixth-floor apartment in West Hollywood. Her death in the fall of 1969 kicked off a protracted public-relations war between Timothy Leary and Art Linkletter, who claimed Leary had "murdered" his daughter through his LSD advocacy.

LSD was still legal in the summer of 1966, when Huston Smith delivered his paper at the University of California. But it would not be for long. Possession of the drug was outlawed under California law on October 6, 1966. Two years later, the drug was banned under federal law. In 1967, in an article published in the journal *Christianity and Crisis,* Smith announced that he was stepping back from his "initial, rather optimistic appraisal of the promise entheogens ['God-enabling' drugs] hold for religion."

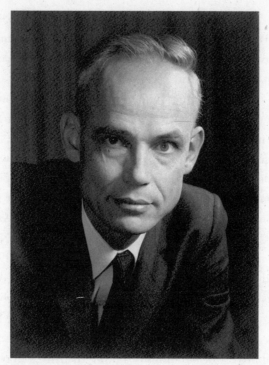

*Huston Smith in the 1960s*

Smith agreed that psychedelic drugs can produce the *experience* of religious mysticism, but he did not find very much evidence that those experiences had the conviction behind them to carry over into the nondrugged state. LSD and other drugs may reshuffle the brain's neurological pathways, stimulate the "euphoria center," and make one feel at one with the world. But that was just not enough to support "the all-too-common, too vague, too uncritical claim that psychedelics expand consciousness.

"Everything seems wonderful because at the moment in question euphoria fills our horizon," he wrote. "The entire world seems wonderful because the world has been collapsed to include only the rose-tinted things we have in mind at the moment."

Smith took greatest exception to Leary's infamous advice that people "turn on, tune in, drop out." That glib message, Smith argued, does not constitute the alternative social vision necessary for the establishment of a viable new religious movement. "If the psychedelic movement were apocalyptic, revolutionary, or utopian, it would present an alternative to the status quo," he wrote. "Being none of these, its social message comes down to 'Quit school. Quit your job. Drop out.' The slogan is too negative to command respect." He also questioned the claim by Leary and others that the psychedelic movement should be treated like any other religious movement, free to consume its mind-bending holy sacrament. Smith saw "no sign of the makings of a church." But Huston went out of his way to avoid directly criticizing Leary, the man who turned him on that memorable New Year's Day in 1961 in Newton, Massachusetts. "The psychedelic movement does have a charismatic leader," Smith wrote, "a man of intelligence, culture, and charm who is completely self-assured and apparently absolutely fearless."

Healer
San Francisco
December 1968

Andrew Weil missed the first flowering of the San Francisco counterculture. He finished his undergraduate work in 1964, and as he'd always planned, he entered Harvard Medical School. He didn't head out to the West Coast until 1968, when he began a yearlong medical residency at Mount Zion Hospital in San Francisco.

"I got to San Francisco a bit late," he would later lament. "The psychedelic era was turning into the amphetamine era."

"Speed Kills" had replaced "Turn On, Tune In, Drop Out" as the received pharmacological wisdom. By 1968, there was a harder edge to the drug scene in San Francisco. Many of the casualties were winding up at the Haight-Ashbury Free Clinic, where Weil worked as a volunteer. Young runaways from across the country came looking for love and peace, but many of them found themselves broke and living on the street, victimized by a variety of sexual and chemical predators.

By the end of his undergraduate years, Andy had stopped experimenting with psychedelic drugs and focused on his academic/medical career. There had been flashes of another reality back during those freshman mescaline trips in Claverly Hall, but Weil was not ready to seriously consider another way of living, another way of experiencing the world. "They were important experiences, but I couldn't deal with them," Weil would later recall. "It threatened my value system and the path I was on. So I really threw myself into being a good Harvard student and getting ready for medical school."

It wasn't until he arrived in San Francisco that Weil felt like he had the space and the time to continue his explorations into other states of consciousness. He reconnected with marijuana and psychedelics. He started dating a nurse at Mount Zion. It was an intense political time. San Francisco was ground zero for the national counterculture. It was such a different cultural scene at Harvard, which was full of intellectuals. In San Francisco, Weil was hanging out with artists and musicians, people he'd never spent time with at Harvard. The years of 1968 and 1969 were the turning point in the life of the bright, ambitious kid from Philadelphia. There was no going home. After that, he tried to go back east, but he felt like a fish out of water.

His time in San Francisco also inspired Weil to look back on what he had done five years earlier to bring down Leary and Alpert. He didn't like what he saw. Weil owed Leary and Alpert an apology, or at least an explanation.

Weil called Leary, and Leary agreed to get together with his old nemesis. "That was a good meeting," Weil recalled. "I told him about the transformations that I'd been through since then, and how I look back on that time. He was easy to be with. It seemed like he'd really let it go."

Weil had a feeling it might be harder to reconcile with Alpert, and he was right. "I told Leary that I wanted to speak with Alpert," Weil recalled, "and he said that would be very difficult."

"Dick is still very angry about the whole thing," Leary replied.

While he didn't know it at the time, Weil was about to go through his own battle with an entrenched bureaucracy—a fight that would be eerily reminiscent of what Leary and Alpert had experienced back at Harvard. Andrew Weil, MD, was about to run up against an administration that did not like his conclusions about a popular street drug.

Talk about karma.


This time the drug was marijuana. It began in December 1968 when Weil authored a report that was published in *Science* magazine. At the time, Weil was only twenty-six years old and still working as an intern at Mount Zion, but the report made headlines across the country.

"The most carefully controlled study to date on the physical and psychological effects of smoking marijuana has concluded that the drug is a 'relatively mild intoxicant with minor, real, short-lived effects,'" the *New York Times* reported. Out on the West Coast, the *San Francisco Chronicle* reported its own interpretation of the study: "Persons who smoke marijuana for the first time do not thereby put themselves on the road to habitual use of the drug, a young scientist declared yesterday."

Weil and two other Boston researchers—a Harvard psychiatrist and a Boston University graduate student—had carried out the study in the spring of 1967, when Weil was still a senior medical student at Harvard. A battery of physiological and psychological tests were given to two groups of college students—nine first-time users of marijuana and eight "chronic users" of the drug. In his report, Weil noted that "it proved extremely difficult to find marijuana-naïve persons in the student population of Boston," adding that "nearly all persons encountered who had not tried marijuana admitted this somewhat apologetically."

At the same time, Weil was careful not to come across as an advocate of marijuana use. Writing later in the *New England Journal of Medicine,* Weil warned that some novice pot smokers may experience mild depression, panic attacks, or "toxic psychosis." Pot smokers who have previously taken LSD, he warned, might have frightening hallucinogenic flashbacks.

In an article published in *Nature,* a British scientific journal, Weil sought to explain why potheads seem so spaced out. After studying tape recordings of stoned subjects trying to verbally express themselves, Weil scientifically confirmed what anyone talking to a stoner at a party knew all too well. "Subtle speech retardation" is caused by a failure of "ultra-short-term memory," Dr. Weil reported. He had discovered that people who are high on pot experience a "simple forgetting of what one is going to say next and a strong tendency to go off on irrelevant tangents because the line of thought is lost."

Those findings were laughable (albeit true) to anyone in the know, but the most important aspect of Weil's marijuana studies was that there were any studies at all. At the time, it was next to impossible to get government permission to legally use marijuana in official research projects. Weil was able to get federal support for his studies. He even got permission to administer marijuana to subjects who had never before taken the drug.

In 1968, the Federal Bureau of Narcotics had cleared the way for him to get research-grade marijuana for his experiments. "I looked over the literature on marijuana," he said. "I couldn't believe there was no experimental basis for statements made about marijuana by pharmacologists and reputable textbooks. It seemed to me the time was ripe to do a study that should have been done thirty years ago."

What inspired Harvard and federal drug agencies to trust Andrew Weil?

Weil believes it was his "reward" for getting the goods on Leary and Alpert back in 1963. "I suspect that the only reason I was allowed to do those marijuana experiments in 1968 was because of the fact that I was the person who wrote the exposé on Leary and Alpert," he said. "One thing I learned was that is the way you advance in that kind of system. I had bought into the value system of that society. Internally, there was this real inconsistency in my life.

I had those mystical [drug-induced] experiences, but to get through medical school I had to stuff all that. It was not until my internship in San Francisco in 1968 that I saw this totally different culture."

In the late 1960s and early 1970s, Weil was living a divided life, not unlike Richard Alpert's experience of being a private homosexual and a public heterosexual. Weil was living half in the straight world and half in the stoned world. In 1970, the director of the National Institute of Mental Health cited Weil's study in his testimony before Congress, saying the young scientist's research was producing "troublesome facts" that "make it impossible to give marijuana a clean bill of health." His conclusion shows how Weil was able to offer something for everyone in his study. Marijuana advocates *and* opponents cited his work, and he was rewarded with a job in the drug-study division of the federal mental-health institute. That prompted him to leave San Francisco in late 1969 and move to Chevy Chase, Maryland.

Weil came to San Francisco to study the hippies, but he'd gone native, and there was no turning back. His transformation can be seen in photographs that ran with newspaper stories about him in the late 1960s and early 1970s. He appeared in December 1968 as a chubby, bald, and clean-shaven physician in a black tie, white shirt, and white lab coat. By the summer of 1971, he'd grown the wild, bushy beard that would become his trademark feature. He'd discarded the coat and tie for faded blue jeans and a work shirt. And he'd slimmed down so much that the *New York Times* observed in a headline that the "Meat-Eating, 230-Pound Doctor Is Now a 175-Pound Vegetarian."

Richard Nixon was president, and Andrew Weil, hippie, would not last long in the drug-study division of the U.S. Public Health Service. He was about to publish his first book, *The Natural Mind: A New Way of Looking at Drugs and the Higher Consciousness,* and let the world know which side he was on. His new bosses did not like his counterculture stance on their "war against drugs."

Neither did Lester Grinspoon, a professor of psychiatry at Harvard Medical School, where Weil had earned his medical degree.

In a scathing review in the *New York Times,* Grinspoon found that Weil presented little evidence to support his basic argument in *The Natural Mind*—that the human desire to get high is as natural as our love of sex and food. "The author attempts to make his arguments irrefutable primarily through his snide dismissal of any facts, experiments, observations or data which do not coincide with his basic premises," Grinspoon wrote. His review found that Weil was "particularly pompous in his ex-cathedra denunciations of all that Western medicine has achieved." Grinspoon dismissed Weil's defense of "stoned thinking" and "straight thinking," taking aim at Weil's warning about how "intellectuals . . . must begin to wake up to the tyranny of the rational (straight) mind."

Grinspoon's harsh critique of Weil's research sounded a lot like Weil's attack on Leary and Alpert's work six years earlier in the *Harvard Crimson.* "The shoddiness of their work as scientists," Weil wrote back then, "is the result less of incompetence than of a conscious rejection of the scientific ways of looking at things."

Decades later, Weil could not look back on that whole period without noting the supreme irony of the whole thing. "I found myself in the same position as Alpert at that point because of my marijuana work," he said. "I was being persecuted for my beliefs."

By the early seventies, Alpert had gone through his own transformation. He had returned from India with an even bushier beard than Weil was sporting and a new name. Weil listened to one of the new spiritual teacher's first lecture tapes, and was blown away. "It had a profound effect on me," Weil recalled. "I realized that I had to make some resolution with the man."

Weil called, but Alpert would not return the call. Richard Alpert may have morphed into the new Ram Dass, but he was still pissed off at the old Andrew Weil.

# CHAPTER SEVEN

# Pilgrimage and Exile

Seeker
Kathmandu, Nepal
December 1967

---

Richard Alpert came to India more as a tourist than a pilgrim. He was traveling with a wealthy friend and patron—a young, retired millionaire Alpert had guided through several psychedelic sessions. They were shocked by the poverty they found in India, and a bit embarrassed by the shiny new Land Rover they'd shipped to Tehran, the starting point for their journey to the mysterious East.

In the four years since he'd been kicked out of Harvard, Alpert had spent much of his time on the lecture circuit, talking about psychedelic drugs and other ways to expand human consciousness. He was burned out. Deep down, he knew he didn't really know what he was talking about, and the hypocrisy of it all was starting to get to him. He went to India not because he thought he was going to find anything. He just didn't know what else to do. He needed a break. He needed a vacation.

Alpert and his friend took some wonderful slides, smoked lots of hash, made tape recordings of Indian music, and then headed up to Kathmandu. By this time, the Nepalese mountaintop was crawling with Western seekers, and one of them, a tall, blond, and beautiful young man from southern California, caught Alpert's eye. His name was Michael Riggs, but he'd been calling himself Bhagavan Das since his encounter with a Hindu guru named Neem Karoli

Baba. Alpert decided that Riggs knew something he didn't. He started following him around India. At first, Alpert had little interest in meeting his new friend's guru. Hinduism seemed like a big, confusing, colorful joke. Alpert was more into Buddhism, a religious philosophy that was neat, clean, and intellectually exquisite. Hinduism seemed a bit sloppy—too garish, gauche, and emotional for his refined taste.

Nevertheless, Alpert agreed to go and at least see Riggs's guru, known to his followers as Maharaji, then took the Land Rover up into the mountains. Alpert's wealthy friend had gone back to the States but had left the luxury car behind for Alpert to use. Riggs was driving and, at one point in the journey, suddenly pulled off the road alongside a little temple, got out of the car, and started running up the hill, crying tears of joy because he knew Maharaji was waiting for them at the top. Alpert went after him, realizing all the way how absurd the situation was. Here was this American guy, barely out of high school, running up to see this Hindu holy man. And here was Alpert, an ex-Harvard professor, running barefoot after him.

They got to the mountaintop, but Alpert was not impressed by what he saw. Maharaji was sitting on a blanket on the ground, surrounded by a small group of Indians. Riggs ran up to him and prostrated himself on the ground, face down, touching the holy man's feet. He was sobbing, and the guru was patting him on the head. Alpert observed the scene, saying to himself, "*No way* am I doing that!"

Maharaji looked up at the skeptical Alpert.

"You came in the big car?"

"Yes," Alpert replied.

"You give it to me?"

Alpert didn't know what to say. First of all, the Land Rover didn't even belong to him, and why in the world should he give it away to this con artist? But before he could answer, Riggs spoke up.

"Maharaji," Riggs said, "if you want it, it's yours."

Alpert was shocked by the offer. "But . . . you can't," he stuttered. "It's not our car."

Everyone started laughing hysterically, and Alpert turned red with embarrassment. *Oh,* he thought, *they're just playing with my head.*

"You made much money in America?" Maharaji asked.

"Yeah," Alpert replied.

"How much do you make?"

"Oh, I don't know, about twenty-five thousand dollars."

"So you'll buy a car like that for me."

Alpert decided to play it cool.

"Well, maybe," he said. "I don't know."

At that point, Maharaji lost interest in this encounter and shooed Alpert and Riggs away. A few hours later, the guru called for Alpert to come and see him.

"You were out under the stars last night?"

"Yeah, I was."

"You were thinking about your mother."

"Yeah," Alpert said, thinking the trickster had made a lucky guess.

"She died last year."

"Yes," Alpert said softly.

Maharaji closed his eyes.

"She got very big in the belly before she died."

"Yeah."

At this point, Richard Alpert's mind began to race. His mother had died six months ago at a Boston hospital after her spleen had enlarged tremendously. How could this guy know that? He hadn't talked to Riggs about any of this.

They sat in silence for a few moments. Alpert started to feel a violent wrenching in his chest, as if a door that had closed long ago was suddenly being forced open. He started sobbing. He wasn't sad. He wasn't happy. About the only words that could describe the feeling were "I'm home."

Alpert went off to spend the night in a nearby house. He couldn't get the encounter out of his mind. Sure, there could have been some way for this strange little man to know about his mother's death. But it didn't seem to matter. The tears were real.

During the night, Alpert remembered that he'd brought a little vial of LSD with him from the States, and had this vague plan that he might offer some to any Indian holy man he might come across to see what kind of reaction they would have to psychedelic drugs. Here was his chance.

Maharaji called Alpert over to see him the next morning, but before Alpert could mention his little experiment, the guru asked, "Where's the medicine?"

"Medicine? What medicine?"

"The medicine, the medicine."

"LSD?" Alpert asked.

"Yes, bring the medicine."

Alpert went over to the Land Rover and pulled out a shoulder bag that contained his medicine kit. He gave the guru three hundred micrograms of LSD—a sizable dose. Alpert spent the whole morning with Maharaji, and nothing happened. Later, the guru told Alpert that LSD could be useful, but it was not true samadhi, that highest state of yogic concentration that the Bhagavad Gita describes as "seeing the self as abiding in all things and all things in the self." The guru said drugs like LSD can allow you to visit the state of consciousness of a saint but won't let you stay there. He used Jesus as an example.

"This medicine allows you the visit of Christ, but you can't stay with him. It would be better to become like Christ than to visit, and this won't do that for you.

"Love," the guru said, "is a much stronger drug than this."

Alpert stayed with Maharaji for eight months for a rigorous meditation regime called *raja* yoga, a method for fostering spiritual evolution. He'd get up each morning at 4:30, bathe in the river in a rite of purification, light candles, chant, and read sacred texts of various faiths, including the Christian faith. Every once in a while he'd look at himself from his old Harvard psychologist state of mind and start laughing. Here he was, a Jew reading the New Testament for the first time, and he was doing it in a Hindu temple in the Himalayas.

Maharaji gave Richard Alpert a new name. He was now known as Ram Dass, which translates into "servant of God."

"Serve people," his new guru told him. "Feed people."

Alpert returned to the States in 1968 and spent two years lecturing as Ram Dass. In Berkeley, an audience of 150 people gathered in a high school auditorium to get their first look at the reincarnated professor. Gone were the horn-rim glasses, clean-shaven face, and slightly nerdy look of the Harvard academic. Ram Dass walked onto the stage bearded and barefoot, wearing a long white robe. A cloud of incense and scented candles drifted across the congregation as he began to speak in a deep, sonorous voice. "Here and now is the existential, holy moment," he said. "You already know that. The only problem is you don't know you know it. That's the Western hang-up—the tremendous need to know, along with not knowing that you know."

To some ears, those were pearls of wisdom. Others heard spiritual clichés and doubletalk—or something you'd hear from someone hopelessly stoned on acid. Outwardly, Richard Alpert was a man transformed, but there were still inner conflicts. He was now wearing the robes of Ram Dass, but he still felt like a phony. He still struggled with his obsessions, especially his bottomless appetite for junk food and anonymous sex. He confessed to a friend that he still had to steel himself against "sneaking out for a pizza or going out to see a pornographic movie." Meanwhile, devotees were lying down to touch his feet, placing their spiritual lives in his hands. Ram Dass charmed them with brutal, self-deprecating honesty. "I don't feel like a holy man," he told them. "I feel like an over-aged hippie, an explorer dilettante." It just made them love him all the more. How humble! How wise!

Ram Dass decided that he wasn't pure enough, and he took off for a second trip to India in November 1970. He wound up at a temple in Bodh Gaya with seventy-five students attending a ten-day Buddhist retreat. Among them were a half-dozen American seekers who would go on to become some of the most popular Buddhist writers and teachers in the United States. Sitting in meditation with Ram Dass were Joseph Goldstein, Sharon Salzberg, Daniel Goleman, Krishna Das, John Travis, and Wes Nisker.

Another seeker at the retreat was Mirabai Bush, a spiritually thirsty grad student from Buffalo, New York. She and her fellow travelers were merely the latest wave of pilgrims to visit the sacred city of Bodh Gaya over the past twenty-five hundred years. They came in the footsteps of original seeker, Prince Gautama Siddhartha, who, according to Buddhist lore, sat under a bodhi tree for three days and three nights until he attained enlightenment.

Mirabai got her first taste of that elusive state about a year before she made her trek to India. She'd been a graduate student at the State University of New York, where she was teaching English to undergraduates and wondering what the hell *that* had to do with everything else that was going on in the world. Protests against the Vietnam War had turned the campus into an armed camp. It seemed like the only real escape from all the turmoil came in the form of one of those tiny tablets of LSD.

Everyone seemed to be taking psychedelics. For many, the experience made the university seem instantly irrelevant. Then a friend who'd been to India and studied with a Tibetan teacher returned to Buffalo with a suitcase full of Tibetan *thangkas*—those wildly colorful, embroidered prayer banners depicting multiarmed Buddhist saints making love or meditating on cushions flying through outer space. What was *that* all about? Something very different was going on out there in the wide, wide world.

Mirabai decided to go for a look, and soon found herself at the temple in Bodh Gaya with Ram Dass and the rest of the dharma bums.

On his first trip to India, Ram Dass had immersed himself in the devotional Hindu practices of his new guru, Neem Karoli Baba. This retreat in Bodh Gaya was led by the Burmese Buddhist teacher S. N. Goenka, who taught a "body scan" meditation technique in which students focus their attention on various parts of their bodies. The practice would later form the basis of the stress-reduction and pain-management work of Jon Kabat-Zinn, the best-selling author and founding director of the Center for Mindfulness in Medicine, Health Care, and Society at the University of Massachusetts Medical School. Ram Dass would also borrow heavily from these Vipassana mindfulness teachings.

The monastery at Bodh Gaya offered a series of ten-day retreats. Some of the Western seekers stayed for months. There was lots of meditation practice, and there was lots of partying. It was one of the first retreats where Goenka had encountered Westerners. These folks were not exactly monks. They would smoke dope in the middle of the retreat and drop acid between sessions. Goenka would give his dharma talk in the evening and go off to bed. Then Ram Dass would start holding court, talking about how the Buddhist teachings related to his Jewishness or his Hindu-ness. Something was brewing in Bodh Gaya, and it was a heady brew.

At the end of one retreat session, a group of Westerners decided it would be fun to go off to Delhi. Magically, a bus appeared with a driver willing to make the trip. So with Ram Dass as ringleader, thirty-four people climbed onto the bus and headed out. Along the way was the city of Allahabad, which hosts a massive spiritual pilgrimage known as the Khumba Mela, which draws sages, sadhus, and saints down from the mountains to ritually bathe in the River Ganges. One of the boys on the bus, Danny Goleman, had been to the festival a few weeks before. Goleman, who would go on to become a noted psychologist, *New York Times* science writer, and best-selling author of *Emotional Intelligence* and other books, thought it would be very cool to make a short detour to the festival site.

"Man, I'd love to have you all see where the Mela was held," he said.

Amid affirmative cheers of "far-out" and "right on," Ram Dass chimed up as the voice of reason.

"Well," he said, "it's kind of late in the day, and we have a small child with us here, and we're all a little tired. It's a long drive to Delhi. Plus, the Mela is over. All we'll see is an empty fairground."

"Yeah," Goleman replied, "but the vibrations will be very beautiful."

"Maybe they will. Maybe they won't. Vibrations are very ephemeral, especially when you're tired. Let's pass this time."

"OK, man," Goleman replied. "Whatever you say."

Then Ram Dass thought about it again. Maybe he was just being an old fart.

"All right," he said. "Let's go."

They got to the junction. The bus driver made a right turn and started heading down a bumpy road. They parked the bus at the bottom of the hill in a deserted fairground. Trash was piled up or blowing across the dusty field. Ram Dass was just starting to think, "So much for good vibrations," when someone yelled, "Look! There's Maharaji!" Everyone piled out of the bus and fell at the feet of Neem Karoli Baba.

"Come," the guru said, "follow me."

Everyone climbed back on the bus and followed a little rickshaw carrying the guru to a house where food and lodging had been prepared for thirty-four people.

Ram Dass could only shake his head. He had no intention of going to see his guru with a bus full of stoned seekers from the States. How did he know they were coming? What is going on here? That just led to more questions for Ram Dass about his own ideas about himself. Who was it sitting in the bus deciding whether we would go to those grounds or not? Who am I? What do I really think the game is? What is behind my decisions? What is ego? What is personality? What is choice? What is free will? What is the possibility of human consciousness? What the hell is going on here, anyway?

Mirabai Bush was equally blown away. Right before the unexpected encounter with the guru, everyone had been sitting around reading the first edition of Ram Dass's counterculture classic, *Be Here Now,* which was put together after Alpert's first trip to India and had just come out in the States. Someone had brought a copy to the monastery at Bodh Gaya, and they had all been passing it around. They'd been reading the stories about this mysterious guru who lives up in the mountains and how you'll find him only if it's in your karma. And there he is. Standing outside the bus! Before she met Ram Dass and encountered his guru, Mirabai had planned to spend about two weeks in India. She wound up staying two years. She took Neem Karoli Baba as her guru and began a lifelong association and friendship with Ram Dass.

They would work together to found the Seva Foundation, which has done charitable works around the world, and coauthor a book titled *Compassion in Action: Setting Out on the Path of Service.* Mirabai would later become the main force behind the Center for Contemplative Mind in Society, founded in 1997 in Northampton, Massachusetts. The center has worked to encourage meditation practice in schools, prisons, and the workplace. And it all traces back to that pilgrimage to India.

Many years later, sitting in her garden in rural Massachusetts, she can only shake her head. "My life completely and utterly changed. It just turned around. Here I was living on the other side of the world. Maharaji was a great gift to us. It's hard to talk about, but he was remarkable. He was simply the embodiment of unconditional love. He radiated love. You felt utterly and totally accepted as you are. I'd never experienced that before. People had loved me, parents and friends, but I'd never experienced anything like it. Everything just shifted. That became the center point. Nothing seemed

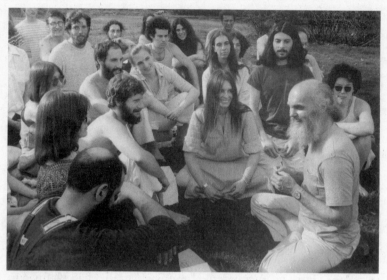

*In this 1975 photo, Ram Dass (bearded, at right) sits in the Cambridge, Massachusetts, garden of David McClelland, his old boss at Harvard. Sitting at his right hand is Mirabai Bush, who met Ram Dass at a retreat in India. (Photo by Peter Simon, courtesy of Mirabai Bush.)*

terrible or serious again after that. There was always that space to return to."

Richard Alpert's psychedelic baptism, followed by his pilgrimage to India, would forever change the way he looked at religion and psychology. "Until psychedelics came along, I'd had negative experiences with religion. I was a member of a conservative temple in Judaism, which never told me about mystical experiences. So I ended up being a social Jew. My father did that too; we had a political and social religion. My view of psychology was also very limited. We treated humans as objects and paid no attention to their inner world. . . . Now I have moved my consciousness past that, I feel that I am merely a cog in a wheel. I'm doing my gig. I'm living my life for God."

## Teacher
## Kyoto, Japan
## Summer 1957

Huston Smith made his first pilgrimage to the Far East ten years before Richard Alpert arrived in India, but both men were in their midthirties when they embarked on their respective quests. Both were young university professors who had climbed the academic ladder, but who were desperately looking for something else. Smith was tired of just writing about satori, the enlightenment experience achieved by some Buddhist practitioners. He'd written enough restaurant reviews of the experience; he desperately wanted a real taste. His first psychedelic drug trip was still three years away. Huston Smith was ready to go halfway around the world for a taste of enlightenment, if that's what it took.

Two visitors to the St. Louis campus of Washington University had inspired a summer trip to Myoshinji Monastery—the Temple of the Marvelous Mind—in Kyoto. The first visitor was D. T. Suzuki, the renowned Zen Buddhist scholar who played a key role in the flowering of Buddhism in the West. Two decades before Smith arranged for Suzuki to visit St. Louis, the prolific Japanese writer had visited England and inspired one of the century's most important reconcilers of East and West—Alan Watts, the influential Anglican/Buddhist writer and lecturer. Watts, who would briefly work with Leary in the early psychedelic research at Harvard, was just a twenty-one-year-old spiritual seeker when he met Suzuki at the World Congress of Faiths in 1936. The second visitor to inspire Huston's journey to Japan was a Japanese priest who was visiting the States on a Fulbright scholarship. He wound up coteaching a course with Smith on Zen Buddhism, and offered some sage advice:

"You will never grasp Zen by the rational mind alone."

Smith decided to go to Kyoto for a summer of meditation.

In Kyoto, he crossed paths with another Zen trailblazer. Gary Snyder—the Beat poet and inspiration for the Japhy Ryder character in Jack Kerouac's novel *The Dharma Bums*—had just arrived in the historic Japanese city. Like Huston Smith and Alan Watts, Gary Snyder had been inspired by the scholarly writings of D. T. Suzuki to make his own pilgrimage to the Zen temples of Kyoto. He would spend most of the next thirteen years in Japan. And while Smith would spend only six weeks at Myoshinji Temple, the experience would have a profound effect on the religion scholar's own spiritual journey.

Through Vedanta, the religious practice Smith embraced after his encounters with Gerald Heard and Aldous Huxley, the freewheeling Methodist had already explored the spiritual disciplines of Hinduism. After returning from Japan, Smith would begin his fifteen-year tenure at MIT, a period when Zen Buddhism was his primary meditation practice. "In switching I don't feel as if I'm deserting Vedanta," Smith told a friend. "Same truth, different idiom."

His native Methodism proved more of a struggle.

At Myoshinji Temple in Kyoto, Smith was placed under the spiritual tutelage of the Zen master Goto Roshi. Smith studiously adhered to the prescribed rituals of the daily visit with Roshi. At precisely 5 A.M., he would slide open the shoji—the door covered with rice paper—bow with palms together, and step into the master's presence. Roshi would be in the opposite corner of the room, seated in his robes on a meditation cushion. Smith would walk slowly along the walls of the chamber, then make a right turn toward the master. On reaching him, Smith sank to his knees and, with his forehead on the straw mat, extended his arms toward his teacher, lifting cupped fingers upward.

At first, the Methodist minister found this practice grating. His Protestant upbringing had admonished him to bow down to neither priest nor king, but there he was—kowtowing to a mere mortal! But after a few days of practice, Smith's disdain for the bowing practice began to dissolve, only to be replaced by another psychological quandary.

Huston's six-week session gave him a chance to try out a variety of Zen techniques. There was the basic practice—periods of sitting meditation punctuated with short meetings with Roshi. Then there was another eight days of looking into the heart and mind. There was also time for Smith to study the English-language manuscripts of the Kyoto branch of the First Zen Institute of America. But the Buddhist practice that almost drove Smith insane was the koan, a seemingly nonsensical riddle designed to snap the student out of his normal way of thinking.

Perhaps the most famous koan is the question, What is the sound of one hand clapping? Smith's koan came from a question that a monk once asked Joshu, a Chinese meditation master from the Tang dynasty.

"Does a dog have Buddha nature?" the Tang monk asked.

"*Mu,*" Joshu replied.

At first, Smith thought he'd gotten an easy one. Everything has Buddha nature. So why not dogs? Then Roshi explained that *mu* is more of a negative response. That puzzled the student. *How can a dog* not *have a Buddha nature,* Smith thought, *when even grass has it?*

Smith spent six weeks kicking that damn koan around in his head, during which time Roshi would give him little hints but never any answers.

"You're a philosopher," Roshi said. "Nothing wrong with philosophy, but philosophy only works with reason. Nothing wrong with reason, but reason only works when it has experience at its disposal. You have reason. Enlarge your experience."

Huston sat on his cushion, trying to stop thinking and start feeling. *"Mu." It's got to have something to do with that damned "mu"! Oops. You're thinking. Stop thinking.* As the session wore on, and the periods of meditation increased, Smith had trouble just staying awake. He was allowed only three and a half hours of sleep a night. Maybe he was getting into an altered state of consciousness, but if so it was because of sleep deprivation, not meditation. What was happening in his mind was more like insanity than enlightenment.

This is not what he read about in all those classic texts describing the experience of satori. Boredom gave way to self-pity, which opened the door to rage.

Two days before the end of the session, he went to Roshi for his daily interview. Their eyes met in a mutual glare.

"How's it going?"

"Terrible," Smith shouted.

"You think you are getting sick, don't you?"

In fact, Huston had been feeling ill. His throat was tight, and he had trouble breathing.

"Yes," he yelled. "I think I'm getting sick!"

Until that point, Smith thought Roshi was taunting him. Mocking him. Suddenly the face of the Zen master softened into a kind of relaxed radiance.

"What is sickness? What is health?" he said. "Put both aside and go forward."

Smith's feeling of rage vanished. He had felt like he was going insane. Now he felt fine. What happened? How did Roshi do that? Did Roshi do that? Huston was asking himself the same kind of questions Ram Dass would ask ten years later when all those little miracles kept happening around his guru.

Smith came to see that Zen meditation and the mysteries of the koan were not simply a rejection of logic and reason. Reason can be useful, he saw, but it is a ladder too short to reach to truth's full heights. It's difficult to even talk about the goals of meditation. The word *zazen* simply means "seated meditation," and that's all you do. You just sit. Some may experience an intuitive breakthrough, seeing into one's true nature. Some may experience satori, a new kind of understanding. Some may just experience frustration and a pain in the neck.

"Just sitting" was a difficult concept for Smith to contemplate. So far, he'd spent his life worshipping at the altar of reason, as an intellectual trying to come to a new understanding of the religious quest. "We in the West," he would later write, "rely on reason so fully that we must remind ourselves that in Zen we are dealing with a perspective that is convinced that reason is limited and must be supplemented by another mode of knowing."

Decades later, Huston still didn't know exactly what happened during that penultimate meeting with Goto Roshi. The Zen master had played him like a violin, stroking his rage and frustration until something snapped. Something happened. It was about feeling, not about thinking. Intuition, not intellect. It had something to do with realizing the limits of the rational mind, something about the union of opposites.

"What I do know is that I have never felt so instantly reborn and energized," Smith would later write. "In that climactic moment I passed my koan, not just theoretically, but *experientially*."

## Healer
### Along the Colombia–Ecuador border
### Spring 1973

Richard Alpert and Huston Smith journeyed to the East on their pilgrimage of self-discovery, but Andrew Weil went off in another direction. He headed south, through Mexico and Central America and into a remote northwestern region of the Amazon rain forest. He was looking for Pedro, a Kofan Indian shaman and healer— not exactly the sort of physician they were turning out back at Harvard Medical School.

Andy was at a turning point in his life. After graduating from Harvard, young Dr. Weil moved out to San Francisco to complete his residency and revel in the Dionysian rites of the Bay Area counterculture. He'd returned to the East Coast for his ill-fated appointment with the drug-study division of the U.S. Public Health Service. He was finishing up his first book, *The Natural Mind,* and he knew that its sympathetic view of the drug culture—the very culture that President Richard Nixon had just declared war against—would undermine his future employment with the government and the American medical establishment. Weil had aligned himself as an outsider, someone on the side of the very people he had worked so hard to bring down a decade before. He was starting to realize how it felt to be Richard Alpert and Timothy Leary.

So, on a rainy night in September 1971, Weil packed up his red 1969 Land Rover and left his home in Sterling, Virginia. It would be a four-year journey.

Richard Alpert and Huston Smith were drawn to the mystical teachings of Buddhism and Hinduism, but Weil was interested in something else. Since his childhood in Philadelphia, when he culti-vated potted plants behind his parent's row house, Andy had shown a fascination with the plant kingdom. As an undergraduate at Har-vard, Weil became a student of Professor Richard Evans Schultes, a pioneer in the field of ethnobotany, which studies the complex relationships between people and plants. Schultes had traveled throughout the Western Hemisphere and done some of the earli-est academic research into the use of the peyote cactus, psilocybin mushroom, and other hallucinogenic plants by indigenous tribes on both continents. Schultes would later coauthor a much-read book with Albert Hofmann, the discoverer of LSD, titled *The Plants of the God: Their Sacred, Healing, and Hallucinogenic Powers.*

Andy Weil was not alone in his fascination with magical plants and mysterious shamans. In the early 1970s, an entire drug-addled generation was enthralled by a series of best-selling books put out by a former UCLA anthropology student. His name was Carlos Castaneda, and he told fantastic tales of his purported apprentice-ship with Don Juan Matus, a Yaqui Indian sorcerer in Sonora, Mexico. The first book began with a disclaimer that the contents are "both ethnography and allegory." Castaneda's readers were never sure how much of his tale was fact and how much fiction. Nor did they seem to care. After all, many of Castaneda's fans had themselves experimented with peyote and magic mushrooms, the very plants that fueled the adventures of the intrepid anthropolo-gist and his trickster teacher. They knew exactly what Castaneda was talking about when he titled his second book *A Separate Real-ity.* They, like him, were convinced that psychedelic insights were "real" in their own way, even if they were based on hallucinations.

The Institute of Current World Affairs, a New York foundation, paid for Weil's pilgrimage. It merely required him to file a few reports and brief monthly newsletters describing his research into the ways different cultures use drugs, plants, and other techniques to achieve altered states of consciousness. Weil was not *just* interested in getting high. He wanted to know what these indigenous healers could teach the medical establishment about health and healing. Weil had begun the 1970s with a freshly minted medical degree from one of the nation's most prestigious medical schools, but he had little interest in the invasive, high-tech treatments that would soon dominate health care in America.

At the same time, getting high *was* part of the research protocol. By the time Weil arrived in the northeastern corner of Oaxaca, Mexico, the locals had grown tired of an endless stream of mushroom-seeking hippies washing onto their shores. They'd had enough of those long-haired seekers with ragged Carlos Castaneda paperbacks in their backpacks. Government troops had even been sent in to clear out the freakish gringos. Weil saw himself more in the tradition of Professor Schultes and Gordon Wasson, the amateur anthropologist who'd tasted the forbidden fungi twenty years earlier and documented his work in *Life* magazine. Weil was able to charm the locals enough to be allowed entry into the home of Julieta, a *curandera,* or healer, who lived in the town of Huautla. Julieta's three-room home, which she shared with her husband and their five children, had stunning views of the steep green peaks of the Sierra Mazateca. Weil was surprised to see that the local healer's pharmacological cabinet contained both a supply of modern antibiotics and a stash of San Isidro mushrooms.

Julieta agreed to lead a traditional mushroom ceremony that night at midnight, after the kids had been put to bed and the house locked up. She set up an altar on a low table in the kitchen that included a framed portrait of San Isidro, a popular Mexican household saint. The *curandera* lit a small charcoal fire to burn two types of incense, a resin similar to frankincense and an aromatic wood called *palo santo*. Julieta purified her face and hands in the smoke, and asked Weil to do the same. Then she lovingly placed two large mushrooms on a little dish and handed them to Weil, who took his first bite. He was surprised how good they tasted, and didn't hesitate when Julieta handed him another dish with seven smaller mushrooms, and then another dish, and another dish, until Weil had eaten about twenty of them. After about a half hour, a feeling of extraordinary contentment settled over the initiate. There was a sense of lightness, of well-being. Julieta knelt before the portrait of San Isidro and thrice repeated the Lord's Prayer. Weil started seeing minor hallucinations, gentle waves of color on all the surfaces in the room. At the *curandera*'s suggestion, Weil went outside to "learn from the moon."

It was dark. The sky was full of stars, but Weil could not find the moon. Then he saw it, low over the western mountains, a silver crescent over a dull gold disk. It was an eclipse! He waited, breathless, as the eclipse progressed to totality. What a spectacle! Then there was the stillness of the night. Such magic!

Weil was to spend one more night at the house. There were some leftover mushrooms, and Julieta suggested that he might as well finish them off. At first, Weil hesitated. It had been so perfect the night before. But then he changed his mind. When else would he have such an opportunity? Julieta performed the same ceremony, but this time the feeling was very different. A heavy fog bank closed in around the house, the temperature dropped, and suddenly nearly everyone in the house was sick. Weil heard crying and coughing from the bedroom. He began feeling sick, then buried in his own fog of depression and isolation. He couldn't sleep. The mushrooms were working against him, not with him. The previous night he had felt like he was at one with the universe. On this night, he felt alone, disconnected from everything around him.

There was a lesson in the experience, one that many psychedelic explorers learn the hard way. As Aldous Huxley wrote two decades before in *The Doors of Perception,* these are powerful, unpredictable substances. Weil had been greedy. He should have trusted his first intuition, which was to honor the initial experience, and not gobble down more mushrooms just because they were available.

Weil's experiences with the Mexican *curandera* were powerful, but the real turning point in his pilgrimage came in South America, on a tributary of the Caqueta River in a remote region of Ecuador. He had heard stories about a Kofan Indian trader named Pedro, who supposedly lived in a hut about a half day's walk into the forest. Weil had already met a number of native healers and shamans on his journey. He was not impressed. Some were drunks; others were obvious con artists. Pedro was supposed to be different, a powerful healer unknown to anyone in the outside world. Weil was searching for something exotic and extraordinary, something worlds away from his ordinary experience. He desperately wanted to find new insight into the *source* of healing power. He wanted to explore the interconnectedness of magic, religion, and medicine.

Pedro was his last hope, and he was not an easy guy to find. Weil parked his Land Rover, traveled by boat to a small frontier settlement, and then found an Indian who took him by canoe to the trailhead that led to Pedro's hut. Weil set out but soon came to a fork in the trail—a junction his guide did not mention. He decided to take the right-hand road. It was the wrong trail. Weil ended up in a dense thicket back at the river. It was a dead end. Weil had a hammock in his backpack and thought about spending the night, but the mosquitoes were eating him alive. Plus, he hadn't brought much food with him. He did have a package of cocoa mix and some dried fruit. He fired up his little backpacking stove, heated up some river water, sat down with his cup of hot chocolate, and pondered his next move.

Wading into the river, he noticed a sandbar upstream, a perch that might give him a better vantage point. It did. He came to a clearing where two rivers joined and spotted a hut in a small

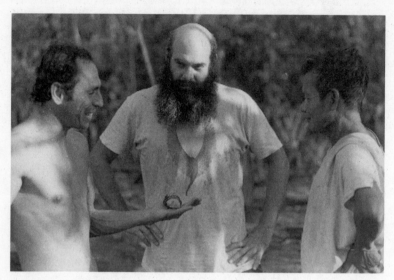

*Andrew Weil, in the early 1970s, on his pilgrimage to South America (Photo courtesy of Andrew Weil.)*

clearing by the river—a thatched hut elevated on stilts, with a crude stairway leading up to a small deck. Weil was ecstatic. He'd found it, and just in time. The sun was going down in a spectacular Technicolor sunset. He ran up to the hut, where he found a young Indian girl, but no Pedro. He'd left ten days ago, she said, and was supposed to be back by now. The girl agreed to let Weil string up his hammock on the deck and pass the night. One night led to two and two nights led to three. Still no Pedro. Weil passed the time lying around, swimming in the river, and reading a Jack London novel he'd brought with him.

Pedro appeared on the fourth day. He turned out to be a serious man in his early forties. He was friendly enough, but he had absolutely no interest in talking to Weil about indigenous healing techniques. He told Weil that he had stopped working as a healer and had become a political activist organizing against an oil company that had come into the region to exploit its rich reserves. Weil spent one more night, then headed back down the trail to his Land Rover and civilization. Weil would spend another year in Colombia, Ecuador, and Peru, but he was done playing the Carlos Castaneda game. Never again, he told himself. Never again would he embark on an arduous journey in search of a man with magical power.

"Pedro taught me that I was looking for answers in the wrong way," Weil would later say. "I did not have to turn away from my own land and culture, my formal education, and my own self to find the source of healing. But I did have to spend those years wandering in order to figure that out."

Trickster
Lausanne, Switzerland
Summer 1971

Timothy Leary had been in jail before, but this time was different. Three Swiss cops had shown up at his apartment in Villars-sur-Ollon, a ski resort in the Bernese Alps, and taken him into custody on an Interpol warrant. Leary had been enjoying a life of exile in politically neutral Switzerland when the long arm of international law reached out and tossed him in the Prison du Bois-Mermet in Lausanne. The cell door slammed shut, and Tim sank into a deep depression. Suicide crossed his mind. He began to cheer up only when one of his Swiss protectors sent over a box of wine and cheese, some books, a typewriter, and several reams of blank paper. After all, Leary *did* have that book to write—a sensational story about his escape from another prison.

Leary had been on the run since September 12, 1970, when he made headlines around the world by eluding his previous captors. The man who told a generation of Americans to "drop out" had been forced to drop off the face of the earth. His new life had begun, and it was a life in exile.

Richard Alpert, Huston Smith, and Andrew Weil left the country on pilgrimages to India, Japan, and Latin America, respectively. Though Leary did visit India in the mid-1960s, that trip was more of a vacation than a pilgrimage. Actually, it was a honeymoon with his third wife, Nena von Schlebrügge, who would soon divorce him. Leary's real "pilgrimage" was the period of his life from 1970 to 1974, when he was either on the run, living in exile, or locked away in prison.

It all began with his dramatic escape from the California Men's Colony, a minimum-security prison outside San Luis Obispo where Leary had been sent after losing an appeal on a 1968 conviction for marijuana possession. He got out by climbing a utility poll, then lowering himself hand-over-hand down a support cable that crossed over the twelve-foot-high cyclone fence. Members of the Weather Underground rendezvoused with the fugitive and stashed him in a camper in nearby Morro Bay. Another team of radicals took Leary's prison clothes and left them in a gas station men's room south of the prison to make it look like he'd headed down to Los Angeles. But Leary headed north, to a safe house in the Bay Area, where he dyed his hair red and shaved some of it off so that he appeared to be a balding man. Timothy Leary was now "William John McNellis," a salesman from Salt Lake City. After hiding out for a week in a farmhouse near Redding, California, Leary made his way down to Utah to meet leaders of the Weather Underground, including Bill Ayers and his wife, Bernadette Dohrn. They created "William McNellis" with a forged birth certificate, Social Security card, and hunting license—papers that required no preexisting photo ID.

Leary then flew off to Detroit, where the task at hand was to obtain a U.S. passport for a guy who did not really exist. Leary, posing as McNellis, walked into the federal building in Detroit with another Weather Underground fugitive calling herself "Aunt Bridget." Standing at a counter beneath a framed portrait of President Nixon, they filled out the passport application, inventing a wife named Sylvia and two lovely children. McNellis was supposed to have a birth certificate and a driver's license to get a passport. He had no photo ID. Leary and his supposed auntie were hoping they could radiate enough down-home charm to get around that requirement.

Leary handed his papers and birth certificate to the woman at the passport counter, who asked him, "Do you have a driver's license, Mr. McNellis?"

"No, I don't," Leary answered, fumbling through his wallet. "I'm afraid I don't drive. Will my Social Security card do?"

"No, sir. I'm sorry. We're supposed to have a photo ID."

"What about your hunting license, dear?" Aunt Bridget suggested.

Leary pulled it out and offered that forged document.

"Well, it has your description, so I guess we can accept this," the clerk said with a smile. "It doesn't have your eye color on here, but I can see your Irish eyes are smiling."

Three hours later, Leary had his passport in hand. And that was all he needed to fool the FBI team at O'Hare International Airport and escape on a flight from Chicago to Paris. His wife, Rosemary, escaped on the same plane, wearing a blond wig and traveling as Mary Margaret McGreedy. From there, the couple flew separately to Algeria, where a new socialist government was offering refuge to a rogue's gallery of leftist fugitives. Leary and his fugitive wife wound up under the protection of Black Panther leader Eldridge Cleaver, who had set up his own "embassy" in a white mansion overlooking the Mediterranean. At first, Leary seemed to revel in his new militant role. He issued a series of manifestos urging the youth of America to revolt. "We have always followed a philosophy of live and let live, love and let love, feel good," Leary wrote. "But never did we suggest or imply that it was our duty or our trip to become masochistic pigeons or sit quietly like good Germans and let a genocidal robot police establishment wipe us out one by one. . . . Anyone who's been through the whole LSD experience with us is an acid revolutionary now. Dynamite is just white light, the external manifestation of the inner white light of the Buddha."

Back in the States, the "peace and love" flock was shocked by Leary's angry messages coming out of Algiers. "One thing we do not need," Richard Alpert quipped, "is one more nut with a gun."

As it turned out, the bomb-throwing incarnation of Timothy Leary did not last long. He and Cleaver soon had a falling-out. The Panthers wanted the lion's share of a $250,000 book advance Leary scored to tell the inside story of his prison escape. They also wanted Leary to renounce the use of LSD. Tim declined, and was put under house arrest for "re-education." Once again, Leary had to escape, but this time it was *from* the Black Panthers. Leary soon came to see Cleaver and his Panther lieutenants as "confused, fearful, uneducated young men who had spent most of their lives in prison or getting there." They spent their time in Algiers "roaring around in their cars and trying to pick up women—a terrible idea in a moralistic Arab land. . . . They were a pathetic joke."

In April 1971, after his falling-out with the Panthers, Leary was given direct protection as a political refugee by the Algerian government, then fled North Africa for the relative comfort of Switzerland. As spring turned to summer in Switzerland, Tim and Rosemary settled into their new lives as political refugees in exile. At first, the Swiss government agreed that the long prison term Leary had been given for marijuana possession was a flagrant abuse of human rights. Leary had been thrown into an American prison because of his political stance, not because he was caught carrying a tiny quantity of pot for his own personal use. But back in the States, the American government was preparing a new case against Leary that focused on his ties to the Brotherhood of Eternal Love, which claimed to be a nonprofit "religious corporation" but looked a lot like a sophisticated drug-smuggling ring. The brotherhood had been created by a group of acid heads who had first crossed paths with Leary back at Millbrook and later opened up a bookstore and head shop in Laguna Beach, California, south of Los Angeles.


Leary's legal troubles began back in 1968, on the day after Christmas, when Tim, Rosemary, and Jack, Leary's son from his first marriage, left the Brotherhood's three-hundred-acre ranch in a

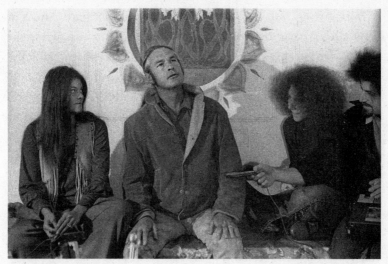

*On May 23, 1969, Timothy Leary looks heavenward as he announces that he is running for governor of California against the incumbent, Ronald Reagan. His wife, Rosemary, sits at the right hand of the counterculture candidate. On his far left, Wes "Scoop" Nisker, then a reporter for KSAN radio in San Francisco, holds a microphone. Shortly after this photo was taken, Nisker dropped acid with Leary while driving him across the Bay Bridge. About a year later, Nisker would run into Richard Alpert at a meditation retreat in India. (Photo by Robert Altman.)*

rural section of southern California. They were headed to Laguna Beach in their blue Ford station wagon when police recognized Leary, stopped the car, conducted a search, and found two half-smoked joints.

At first, Leary's arrest didn't slow down his whirlwind appearances as the trickster of the stoner counterculture. Five months later, in May 1969, Leary announced that he was running for governor of California. At a press conference in Berkeley, as police and demonstrators battled over a piece of university-owned land that had been christened "People's Park," Leary outlined his vision for the Golden State, sitting in the poster-festooned offices of the *Berkeley Barb,* a leading underground newspaper. "Helicopters would not be spraying down war gas," he said, "but love gas and flowers."

Wes "Scoop" Nisker, who would soon meet Richard Alpert at a Buddhist retreat in India, covered the Leary announcement for KSAN, the alternative FM radio station in San Francisco. After the Berkeley press conference, Nisker offered Leary a chance to directly address the people of the Bay Area from the KSAN studios. Scoop even offered to drive Leary from Berkeley to San Francisco. Leary accepted, and on the way to the city, Leary turned to Nisker.

"Hey, man, I've got some acid here and I was going to drop," Leary told his driver. "You want some?"

Nisker wasn't really in the mood for an LSD trip. After all, he was in a car and heading toward the Oakland–San Francisco Bay Bridge. Then Scoop started thinking to himself. *Well, the guy is the "high priest of LSD." What else can I do? When else am I going to get a chance like this?* So, Nisker dropped the acid. By the time they got to the radio station Scoop was so stoned he couldn't put two words together. But Leary sat down behind the microphone and just let out all this beautiful, flowing prose. He was his usual glib, funny self. Nisker was melting into the floor, mumbling to himself. But there was Leary, totally in charge of himself—so charismatic, so facile. What a performance!

Just three days later, Tim and Rosemary Leary were in Montreal, seated at the foot of John Lennon and Yoko Ono's bed for the iconic recording of the sixties anthem "Give Peace a Chance." Tommy Smothers sat next to Leary, strumming the guitar. Lennon returned the favor by writing a song in honor of Leary's run for governor. It was titled "Come Together" and was released in September 1969—the first song on *Abbey Road,* the last album the Beatles started recording before their breakup.

Later that fall, Leary appeared as a defense witness in the conspiracy trial of the "Chicago Seven," who stood accused of starting a riot outside the Democratic Party's 1968 presidential nominating convention. In December 1969, the pied piper of psychedelia ended the year and the decade with an appearance at the infamous free concert the Rolling Stones held at Altamont Speedway east of San Francisco. Leary blamed the violence that marred the concert on the type of intoxicants consumed. "The drugs most on display at Altamont, particularly around the bandstand, were not psychedelic drugs but speed, smack, and booze," he explained.

Woodstock and Altamont would go down in the sixties iconography as the Jekyll and Hyde of the counterculture decade. As the sixties drew to a close, there was a harder edge to the drugs, and to the entire scene. There seemed to be more war than peace, more hate than love. Martin Luther King Jr. was dead, and the Black Panthers were on the rise. The Human Be-In was a fading memory, and the Weather Underground were throwing bombs and making headlines. Richard Nixon was elected president, and then the Beatles broke up.

For Timothy Leary, the close of the sixties was the beginning of a long downhill slide. In February 1970, an Orange County jury found Tim, Rosemary, and Jack Leary guilty of marijuana possession. Superior Court Judge Byron McMillan, who was appointed by Governor Ronald Reagan, the man Leary was running against for governor, sentenced Leary to ten years in prison for possession of two roaches. Leary still faced sentencing on a federal pot-smuggling charge stemming from his 1965 arrest in Laredo, Texas. U.S. District Judge Ben Connally, the brother of Texas Governor John Connally, who had been injured in the 1963 assassination of President Kennedy, sentenced Leary to another ten years in prison.

So, as the new decade began, the forty-nine-year-old Leary faced the possibility of spending the next twenty years in prison. It looked like Timothy Leary would finally fade from the public eye, but the trickster would not be silenced. His September 1970 prison escape, and his subsequent reappearance at the Black Panthers' "government-in-exile" in socialist Algeria, showed the world that he had a few more tricks up his sleeve. Suddenly, he was more infamous than ever—on the front page of newspapers around the world.

That was the good news. The bad news was that Leary was back behind bars. It was the summer of 1971, and it looked like

Leary might be spending the rest of the year at Bois-Mermet Prison in Lausanne. His situation was further complicated because he had signed away most of his book advance to his latest agent and protector, a mysterious French millionaire named Michel-Gustave Hauchard. According to Leary, Hauchard was an embezzler and arms merchant wanted by the French government and now living in Switzerland in luxurious asylum. Hauchard offered a life-style Leary could appreciate, especially after those brutal months in North Africa with the Black Panthers. In Switzerland, there were limousines, fine restaurants, endless champagne, fine Cuban cigars, and an assortment of lovely escorts. Hauchard set Tim and Rosemary up in Villars-sur-Ollon, explaining that it was his "obligation as a gentleman to protect philosophers." He told Leary not to worry about the Swiss police. "The police are no problem to me," he said. "I have a dozen of them on my payroll."

Hauchard's connections were apparently not good enough to keep the Swiss police from tossing Leary into the Prison du Bois-Mermet. Or maybe they were. One account of this chapter in the Leary saga contends that it was Hauchard who arranged for Leary to be taken into custody—a trick designed to get him to focus on that book he had to write. Either way, the mysterious Frenchman was kind enough to treat Leary to a series of care packages. In addition to the typewriter, wine, cheese, and reams of stationery, Leary enjoyed French salami, Swiss chocolates, shredded lobster, and a carton of Gitanes cigarettes.

While Hauchard tried to keep Leary as happy and produc-tive as possible, Rosemary solicited the aid of Allen Ginsberg to circulate a petition calling on the Swiss government to free Leary from prison. The petition, delivered to the Swiss consulate in San Francisco on Bastille Day, July 14, 1971, called on the government to "grant our fellow author philosopher safe political asylum to complete his work." Signers of the document included Ken Kesey, Lawrence Ferlinghetti, Alan Watts, Anaïs Nin, and Laura Huxley, the widow of Aldous. Tim was released two weeks later.

Leary was free, but his life was going nowhere. His marriage to Rosemary was on the rocks. A group of hardcore drug users from California had shown up in Switzerland. Leary went into a downward spiral and briefly added heroin to his pharmacological routine. His estranged wife thought he'd finally lost his mind.

At the same time, the Swiss government rejected a request from the U.S. government that Leary be extradited back to the States. At least he didn't have to worry about the immediate prospect of getting tossed back in jail. But the Swiss government also denied Leary's request for permanent political asylum and said he had to be out of the country by October 31, 1972. Leary had a year of breathing room, but he still had a book to write. Now that he was free, there were way too many distractions, most of them involving sex, drugs, and rock 'n' roll.

Michel-Gustave Hauchard, who stood to make a lot more money than Leary from the book about Leary's prison escape, agreed to import a ghostwriter from Great Britain. His name was Brian Barritt, and his arrival was a mixed blessing. Barritt was a skinny, wide-eyed freak who'd probably taken as much LSD over the past decade as Timothy Leary had consumed. And Brian was even more of a party animal than Tim. But Barritt was also a disciplined writer. Amid all the partying, they actually got the project done. Mostly, they just sat around and talked. Barritt wrote most of the book.

Bantam Books printed twenty-five thousand paperback copies of *Confessions of a Hope Fiend,* releasing the title on July 1, 1973. Michel-Gustave Hauchard held the copyright. Unlike most of Leary's other books, it was never reprinted.

Leary had a few more months to enjoy life in Switzerland, and to plan his next move. He had several meetings with Albert Hofmann, the chemist who had discovered LSD in his Basel lab during World War II. They met for the first time over lunch at the snack bar at the Lausanne train station. Later, the Swiss scientist showed Leary the route of Hofmann's famous bike ride from the Sandoz lab—the scene of the world's first LSD trip.

Hofmann had a love/hate relationship with Leary. He publicly chastised the Harvard researcher for encouraging young people to dabble indiscriminately with the drug. "In the beginning, Albert hated him," said Dieter Hagenbach, a Swiss publisher who knew both men. "Then people began telling Hofmann that if LSD hadn't spread all over the world, the sixties wouldn't have happened and you would not have become the person you are now—the famous Albert Hofmann. Later, during their meetings, they had a great time together. They were fascinated by each other. Albert and Timothy had completely different lives, but they were both great lives. He had discovered the most potent substance on this planet, and Leary let the world know about it. They were like the father and the son. LSD needed Father Albert, but it also needed the son."

Among the visitors who stopped by to pay their respects to Leary over that final summer in Switzerland was Richard Alpert. He arrived at the Leary chalet in his new incarnation as Ram Dass, on his way back to the West from his second pilgrimage in India. On the day Ram Dass showed up, Tim and some friends were getting together to drop acid. Ram Dass was not feeling too good, still recovering from a bout of "Delhi belly," but he joined in by taking a little hash oil. Alpert was starting to put the drug scene behind him, and these guys were hard-core. Ghostwriter Barritt looked particularly wasted.

Timothy Leary had long ago warned the youth of America to stay away from heroin. LSD and marijuana would get you high; heroin would only drag you down. But in the late summer of 1972, with Rosemary gone and his future prospects dim, Timothy Leary turned to smack. It didn't help that he'd been hanging out with Keith Richards, the notorious guitarist for the Rolling Stones. The Stones were in Switzerland in 1972, recording *Exile on Main St.* Leary was living in exile, but Main Street seemed worlds away.

"Rosemary's departure left me desolate," Leary would later explain. "After two years of prison and exile I was cut off from American contacts. No sense of mission, no source of income. Everywhere I went that summer I heard the low-down beat of the Stones celebrating Sister Morphine and Brown Sugar, Mick singing about his basement room and his needle and his spoon, wailing the profound philosophic thought of the season: 'I stuck a needle in my arm. It did some good, it did some harm.'"

Brian Barritt was ready with the needle and the spoon. One of Barritt's friends, a stewardess with Swissair, showed up at the house with a large stash of pure heroin that she'd just smuggled in from Beirut. Leary remembers Barritt shaking his head after shooting up, as he prepared Tim's first needle, mumbling something about how he'd "hate to be known as the person who got Timothy Leary hooked on heroin." That said, he stuck the needle in Leary's arm and pushed the plunger. Leary felt the warm flash of euphoria, a few minutes of wonder, and relaxed into nods of bliss. Then he fell into a heavy sleep.

# CHAPTER EIGHT

# After the Ecstasy . . . Four Lives

Healer
Vail, Arizona
November 2007

---

Andy Weil hops out of the shower, tosses a blue terry-cloth bathrobe over his sweatpants, and walks out as the sun rises over his ranch in southern Arizona. Weil is now sixty-five years old and has, by most measures, lived a very successful life. He has published ten books, several of them best sellers. He's done two PBS series, *Dr. Andrew Weil's Guide to Eating Well* and *Dr. Andrew Weil's Healthy Aging.* *Time* magazine put his face and his Santa Claus beard on its cover *twice* over the last decade, *and* named him one of the twenty-five most influential people in America.

For years, he was the organic thorn in the side of the American medical establishment. Now, Andrew Weil, MD, has a prestigious post as the founding director of the Center for Integrative Medicine at the University of Arizona College of Medicine and is setting up similar programs at medical schools across the country.

Weil's Internet-based business, Dr. Weil's Marketplace, helps fund these projects. Consumers of natural living can shop online for an array of Weil-endorsed products, including Dr. Weil for Origins Plantidote Mega-Mushroom Face Cleanser, Weil By Nature's Path Organic Banana Manna Pure Fruit and Nut Bars, Weil By Nature's Path Organic Chocolada Almond Hot Oatmeal, Weil's Wild Alaskan Sockeye Salmon Sausage, Weil for Tea Oolong Shot, the Pro Juice Extractor by Dr. Weil, Dr. Weil's 12″ Wok, and Dr. Andrew Weil's Mindbody Toolkit. That's all on top of a lucrative business selling vitamins and other dietary supplements. In 2008, these products provided about $650,000 in profits for the foundation that supports Weil's integrative-medicine projects.

His 120-acre ranch sits on the edge of Saguaro National Park, just off the Old Spanish Trail. Visitors must traverse a bumpy dirt road through this stark but stunning desert landscape before arriving at a shady oasis of cypress and pine. Weil has been living in the southern Arizona desert since 1973, when his car broke down on the way back from his pilgrimage across Latin America. He's called this circa-1924 ranch house his home since he bought this property in the mid-1990s, just as his breakthrough book, *Spontaneous Healing,* was settling in for its long ride at the top of the *New York Times* best-seller list. Weil's eight books have sold more than six million copies. His newsletter has more than one hundred thousand subscribers, and millions more have checked out his Web site. Dr. Weil has become CEO of alternative medicine in America, the guru of natural living. The ambitious freshman has become "Dr. Weil, Your Trusted Health Advisor."

Weil's attempts to find a wife and raise a family have not been so successful. He remained unmarried until he was forty-seven years old. In 1990, he married Sabine Kremp, a former divorce mediator and massage therapist. They had a daughter, Diana, and tried to blend that family with three older children from Kremp's previous marriage. For a while, the family seemed to be working—at least on the surface. *People* magazine profiled Weil and his family in a 1995 article and found what seemed like domestic bliss. "Dr. Andrew Weil's house in Arizona teems with life," *People* reported. "There are four kids, three dogs, a cockatiel and Coca the macaw, who chirps 'Hello!' to visitors and shrieks 'Ouch!' when his master sprays him with water to simulate his native rain-forest habitat."

Weil suddenly found himself with a wife and four kids—just as his long-simmering career was coming to a rapid boil. Just twenty months after the family was profiled in *People* magazine, the marriage went up in flames. Weil had become a national media celebrity. Everyone wanted a piece of him. In addition to being his wife, Sabine Kremp was Weil's business manager. "Running this empire," Kremp said, "has been tough." Andy and Sabine divorced in 1998. Kremp moved to Utah with the kids. A year later, Weil was just starting to come out of the emotional turmoil. It had been too much for him, trying to blend his wife's family with their new daughter. "From my point of view, it was the difficulty with the stepkids," he said. "It didn't help that it happened during this big explosion of publicity."

*Explosion* is the right word. Why did his career suddenly take off? Weil had been saying the same thing since the 1970s. Weil didn't change. America changed. Sometime in the 1990s, American culture caught up with the sixties counterculture. The counterculture became the culture. Yoga became big business. Meditation is prescribed by the family doctor. Supermarkets stock organic produce and homeopathic cures. The Rolling Stones provide the soundtrack for computer advertisements, and Dennis Hopper promotes corporate retirement funds on network TV.

Looking back on it all, Weil sees a direct connection between his experiences on psychedelic drugs and his later career in holistic health. "Those experiences showed me that what's inside your head is connected to what's outside your head and that you change things outside by working on things inside," he said. "And there is a clear application to health there. State of mind, belief, and expectations absolutely influence health and the course of illness. In those days, that kind of thinking was pretty much out of the mainstream. Now that has really changed."

That's true, but there was more to Weil's meteoric rise than the culture catching up. Something else changed in the selling of Andy Weil. The marketing changed. Weil had been a niche author. Deciding it was time to roll himself out to a wider audience, Weil switched agents. He had been represented by Lynn Nesbit, a New York literary agent, who infamously quipped, "If Andy Weil really wants to make it, he's got to shave off his beard." Andy Weil loves his beard. If he could, he would trademark that, too. Weil's new agent, Richard Pine, declined to take credit for his client's new-found audience. "Like many truly innovative people, he was just ahead of his time," Pine said. "In 1995, consumers and the mass media were ready to hear and read what he had to say. It wasn't me that made him viable in a big way. It was the crisis in mainstream medicine."

Mainstream medicine fought back. Leading the attack was Dr. Arnold S. Relman, the former editor of the prestigious *New England Journal of Medicine*—a man who helped Weil learn the physician's trade when Relman taught at Harvard Medical School back in the 1960s. Relman wrote a lengthy critique of Weil's work and had it published in the *New Republic*. He said Weil's endorsement of herbal supplements, claims of miracle cures, and reliance on various "mind-body" exercises were often based on "notions totally at odds with science, common sense, and modern conceptions of the structure and the function of the human body." Weil and other practitioners of alternative medicine "do not appear to recognize the need for objective evidence, asserting that the intuitions and the personal beliefs of patients and healers are all that is needed to validate their methods."

Relman conceded that some of Weil's criticisms of mainstream medicine were valid, and helped explain the public's embrace of diet supplements, meditation techniques, herbs, homeopathic cures, and Chinese healing techniques such as acupuncture. It is true, Relman wrote, that doctors are too quick to resort to surgery, costly technology, and potent drugs when simple, less invasive methods could work just as well. He also speculated that Weil's vigorous endorsements of healing herbs "stem from his earlier training in botany and his long interest in the psychedelic properties of plants.

"Weil would seem at first to be ideally suited to be a leader of the alternative medicine movement at this juncture," Relman continued. "He is articulate, self-assured, intellectually nimble—and wonderfully ambiguous. Ambiguity, after all, should be helpful to those who would defend systems of healing that are based on irrational or non-existent theories and are supported by no credible empirical evidence."

Weil is sensitive to such criticism, and responded in 2005 in his next book, another national best seller, titled *Healthy Aging*. He points out that he does change his recommendations on the value of various supplements by keeping up with current scientific research, and that he has always favored greater government regulation of dietary supplements. Weil and Relman sparred for a year or two, but Andy Weil just kept enlarging his audience and expanding his market, selling more books and products on his burgeoning Web site. As the new millennium began, Weil took to endorsing everything from gourmet olive oil to his own line of cookware. Ten years after the 1995 release of his breakthrough book, Weil was back on public television to promote *Healthy Aging*. The children of the sixties were heading into their golden years, and Andy Weil was right there with them. The guy who once offered advice on how to find the most potent magic mushrooms was now peddling tiny bottles of Plantidote Mega-Mushroom Face Serum, guaranteed to bring "renewed radiance and clarity" to the wrinkled skin of aging hippies.

Here, on this November morning in the dry Arizona desert, Weil seems happy, even ready to slow down a bit. On a clearing in the scrubby desert, not far from his office in the old horse barn, Weil has constructed a stone labyrinth, a meandering circular path used for periods of walking meditation and reflection. In recent years, these pathways of spiraling concentric circles—patterned after one built into the floor of Chartres Cathedral in France more than eight centuries ago—have been popping up in church parking lots and New Age retreat centers across the country and around the world. Weil's labyrinth is a simple one, with the pathway outlined with stones laid out on a round patch of the desert floor. Weil's ranch foreman has ended his tour here, explaining that this simple design replaced a more elaborate labyrinth that was washed out by a flash

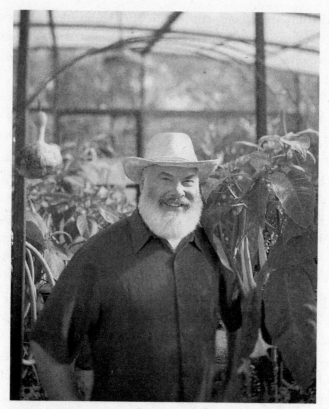

*Andrew Weil at his Arizona ranch (Photo courtesy of Weil Lifestyle, LLC.)*

flood that swept over the property in the summer of 2006, causing significant damage and washing away books, records, papers, and other items Weil had collected over the course of his life.

Life on the ranch was just getting back to normal, as was the rest of Weil's existence. He had just built a luxurious getaway house up in British Columbia, on Cortes Island, where Weil can escape during the blistering days of summer. "It's where I go to disconnect," he explained.

It's been more than four decades since Weil first made headlines with his damning exposé of Timothy Leary and Richard Alpert. Weil is not proud of what he did back then. He feels like he made up with Leary before The Trickster's 1996 death. One turning point came in 1983 when Leary, the old LSD guru and sixties relic, was coming out with an autobiography, appropriated titled *Flashbacks*. The publisher had sent a galley of the new book to Weil's office in Tucson, hoping for a favorable blurb from the man who'd replaced Leary as the go-to guy on mind-altering drugs. "*Flashbacks* is filled with good stories, celebrities, zaniness, and solid information about the psychedelic revolution of the sixties and the man who was its chief proponent," Weil wrote.

It was a nice blurb. But it would take more than a literary endorsement to mend the fences with Richard Alpert. Weil has made several attempts over the years to apologize and reconcile with Ram Dass—the man who had a lot to do with Weil getting interested in yoga and meditation. Weil did a benefit to help raise money for Ram Dass and the medical expenses he incurred following a severe stroke in 1991. They later met in Hawaii, where Weil was giving a talk. Ram Dass showed up. On the surface, it looked like they had reconciled, but Weil kept hearing from mutual friends that Ram Dass was still upset about the way Weil went after him back at Harvard.

"There's still some stuff there that he hasn't expressed to me," Weil said. "He's a complicated guy."

Seeker
Maui, Hawaii
January 2008

Ram Dass struggles to get out of his wheelchair and into the over-stuffed recliner. It's been more than a decade since the stroke, and he still has trouble talking. The right side of his body remains paralyzed. There have been other medical problems that almost did him in. He says he's come to Maui to die.

He's spent much of his life talking about his transformation from Richard Alpert to Ram Dass, but there are parts of the story he has tried to keep to himself. At first, he doesn't really want to talk about what happened with those two undergraduates back at Harvard, Ronnie Winston and Andrew Weil. Something inside him still tightens up with the mere mention of the name Andrew Weil.

"It's a complicated relationship," he says.

It has been a tough ten years for The Seeker. The struggle began one evening in February 1997. Ram Dass was at his home in Marin County, just north of San Francisco, working on his next book, tentatively titled *Conscious Aging,* when he fell into a dream. He dreamed that he was a very old man with failing eyesight and failing legs. In the dream, one of his legs was numb, and he fell over when he got up to answer a phone call. "R.D.? Are you there?" The man in the dream mumbled some incoherent answer. The guy on the other end of the phone, an old friend from Santa Fe, realized that this was not a dream. This was real, and something was very wrong with Ram Dass. He called one of Ram Dass's secretaries, who lived nearby. She rushed over, found him on the floor, and called an ambulance. He had suffered a massive cerebral hemorrhage. Doctors gave him a 10 percent chance of survival.

Ram Dass survived, but it hasn't been easy. For years, he had been the helper. He even wrote a book called *How Can I Help?* Now he was the one who needed help. He had spent years working with the dying, hearing stories of great visions and grand epiphanies that come at the end. He was writing a book on aging, but until the stroke, he didn't think of himself as old. He was a vibrant sixty-six-year-old guy tooling around in his MG—the life of the party. But the stroke showed him—once again—how God has a strange sense of humor, and that he still had some work to do on himself. He'd come face-to-face with death and felt nothing—no long tunnels, no white light. "Here I am, 'Dr. Spiritual,' and in my own death I didn't orient toward the spirit. I flunked the test."

Those who know Ram Dass well say his stroke, as hard as it was, may have been the best thing to happen to him. He seems more human now. He's got less of an edge. He seems to have mellowed out. Amid all the talk of compassion and bliss, there was always a slightly angry, snappish side that would reveal itself from time to time. "As he gets older, he gets sweeter and more loving," observed his old friend from India, Mirabai Bush. "The stroke allowed him to let go of a lot of his critical judgments of people."

During much of the 1980s and 1990s, Ram Dass lent his name and energies to a series of charities and volunteer projects. In the process, he became one of the most sought-after speakers on the New Age conference, workshop, and lecture circuit, where he was known for his ability to convey mystical ideas with lucidity, humor, and grace.

Many of those in his audience were aging baby boomers still trying to make sense of the soul-shattering, consciousness-raising experiences they had on psychedelic drugs way back in the 1960s. Ram Dass inspired many of them to go beyond the revelatory insights that psychedelic drugs can provide, and pursue a less dangerous, more life-affirming spiritual practice. "People's minds were blown, shall we say, for lack of a better phrase," Mirabai recalls. "He was the only one who really could explain and guide people into what was happening from a psychological perspective. He knew psychology and he knew psychedelics, and he was just the best at being able to put that together to know what was going on. Without that we could have lost a lot more people. People were so grateful. It was just the right moment. He had the right intelligence and background to work with it—and he was very charismatic."*

Ram Dass never forgot the mission given to him in 1967 by his Indian guru, the late Neem Karoli Baba, to love God and serve people. He was the founding inspiration behind several ongoing charitable concerns, including the Seva Foundation, which has

---

*Among those inspired by Ram Dass was Wayne Dyer, the best-selling self-help writer and public-television guru. "To me, Ram Dass was and is the finest speaker I have ever heard," Dyer wrote. "He was my role model on stage. . . . He was the voice of Applied Spirituality—his life was the model."

worked for three decades on health and welfare projects in India and Guatemala and on Native American reservations in the United States. Mirabai Bush, one of the cofounders of Seva, said there were many clashes on the Seva board over whether the organization should take a more political, activist stand on social issues. Ram Dass wanted to stick to straight charity. "He was critical of those of us leaning more toward social action," she said. "He was often cranky about it. He was a bad boy a lot. He'd say, 'That's it. This is my last meeting!' Then everything would stop while we dealt with that. Other people were angry about injustice, and he'd struggle with that. He'd say, 'You're just caught up in your anger.' He wasn't always very understanding about *why* people were angry."

Social and political activism was never a priority with Leary or Alpert. They were not out marching to stop the war in Vietnam, nor even talking about it. In fact, they helped set the tone for the political disconnectedness of much of the human-potential and New Age movements, whose politics—or lack of it—were reflected in that line from the Beatle's tune "Revolution." If you want true freedom, the song suggests, "You better free your mind instead."

Not surprisingly, this upset many of Leary and Alpert's would-be allies in the more radical wing of the counterculture. Sixties political activist Michael Rossman, one of the leaders of the 1964 Free Speech Movement at UC Berkeley, remembers with disdain an evening in the 1970s when Ram Dass came to the Berkeley campus to address the next wave of Cal undergraduates. Rossman could hardly believe his ears when the professorial guru started talking about politics. "I know there's a lot of oppression and injustice in this country," Ram Dass told the crowd. "But we must remember to be grateful for the most important thing, that a meeting like this is allowed to go on here." And then, Rossman recalled, Ram Dass "goes on with this song about the gods protecting us, and I wonder what function and whom this meeting serves, and feel a chill wind rising in this closed room of the spirit."

In the early years, other Seva leaders wanted to take a more political approach to helping the poor, but they knew they couldn't survive without Ram Dass. He was the organization's superstar and fund-raising magnet. "Ram Dass always struggled over money, but he raised so much of it over his lifetime. And he gave it all away," Mirabai Bush recalled. "When he had his stroke, he was broke. He had nothing. His father was a big fund-raiser, so he knew how to do it. He brought his upwardly mobile, Jewish, upper-middle class set of values around money, but never really knew what to do with it."

Ram Dass also struggled with all of the fame and adoration of a generation that wanted to put him on a pedestal. "When we first came back from India, he couldn't walk down the street. People were just coming from all over the place," Mirabai recalled. "People would deify him. He didn't want it. It gave him the creeps, but it's hard to keep straight about all that when people are constantly telling you how great you are. The best part of him didn't want it, but it was hard for him to manage."

One of the more appealing aspects of Ram Dass's story is the way he never quite seems to believe his own insight. Paradoxically, this self-deprecation only makes him *more* believable. "You see, I am so used to conning people. I'm used to being so charming and charismatic," he told an interviewer in 1985. "People always want something from me. It can just be a smile, but they want something. . . . You don't know how desperately I wanted that experience of not being able to charm somebody. Because the minute I charm, that paranoia begins. They don't really know the real me."

In 1991, Ram Dass came up with a rather creative way to remind his fellow seekers that true spiritual sustenance requires one to look outside oneself. To encourage "compassion in action," Ram Dass hosted a series of events at the Scottish Rite Temple in Oakland, California. More than a thousand people—most of them white and middle class—signed up for a ten-week experiment called "Reaching Out," a kind of giant support group to foster community service. Participants paid one hundred dollars and then agreed to engage in weekly acts of volunteerism, such as helping out in soup kitchens or working with the sick and dying. Then they discussed their experiences in small group meetings and completed weekly homework assignments of "inner work" and journal writing. Each week, under the gaze of television lights and cameras recording the proceedings for later broadcast, they gathered in the ornate Oakland auditorium. Ram Dass, microphone in one hand, prayer beads in the other, ventured into the audience like a consciousness-raising Oprah, searching for stories about the spiritual overtones of volunteerism. "You know," he said, "this kind of work is far more than 'doing good.' When it's done with a good heart, it's unclear at the end of the helping act who is the helper and who is the helpee."

In some ways, Ram Dass always seemed more like just another seeker on the path, less like some all-knowing guru. Like many in his generation, and the next, he stumbled along the way, and was always ready to admit his failings. Looking back on his life, he confesses that he was always more comfortable playing the loyal lieutenant, the number-two guy. He did that with Timothy Leary. He did it with Neem Karoli Baba. He did it with Chögyam Trungpa Rinpoche, the popular Tibetan Buddhist teacher and founder of the Naropa Institute, who tried to take Ram Dass under his wing. And he did it at least one other time, with some embarrassing results. In the winter of 1974, shortly after the death of Neem Karoli Baba, Ram Dass fell under the spell of a lady named Joya, a spiritual channeler living in New York City. He devoted himself to her and her teachings for more than a year. He would eventually denounce her as a fraud and write a long apologetic article about the experience. He published it in *Yoga Journal* under the headline "Egg on My Beard."

Ram Dass doesn't want to be worshipped, but he wants to be loved. He wants to be known. About five years after his stroke, film director Mickey Lemle released an intimate documentary about Ram Dass. It was a fine movie, but there was something missing. Despite all its intimacy, the film never points out that Ram Dass is gay. Part of that is the subject's fault. "I've had a hard time getting my homosexuality into my drama," he said. "Most of my friends don't like that I'm homosexual. They dissuade me from coming

out. They feel people would have attitudes, would be put off by
it." Ram Dass loved the film's depiction of his struggle with aging,
sickness, and death, but he said he was sorry that the film sanitized
his life. He said he didn't like the way it portrayed him as a hippie
saint.

Over the years, Ram Dass has avoided any detailed discussion of
his own sexuality—with a few notable exceptions. In the 1980s, he
would talk about himself more as a bisexual than as a homosexual.
Here's his answer to an interviewer who asked him, "Do you feel
it's significant that you're not married?"

"Sure it's significant that I'm not married," he replied. "I mean,
I love children and love women and I would like to be married in
some ways. And then in some ways I wouldn't. I live with a woman
and I live with a man and everybody knows everybody and it's all
wonderful. I don't live with them together. They live in different
parts of the country. And I don't live with them on a regular basis
but we are extremely close and trusting and true and we are spiritual companions and there is also physical intimacy."

Working with AIDS patients in the 1980s inspired Ram Dass to
speak out a little more about his own sexual journey. Then, in the
early 1990s, a few years before his stroke, he sat down for a detailed,
almost confessional, interview about his sexual past. He talked
about how in his college years he began having sexual encounters
with men in parks and public bathrooms. He talked about the size
of his genitalia. "I was confused," he explained. "Later, when I
moved to California to do postgraduate work at Stanford, I started
to get more involved in gay life in San Francisco. I've only roughly
estimated, sometimes to just blow people's minds, but I'm sure I've
had thousands of sexual encounters. It was often two a night. Then
I returned east as a professor at Harvard and continued to have this
incredible sexual activity. But I always had a woman as a front to go
to faculty dinners and things like that."

He remained confused about his sexuality after his return from
India. One day, he found himself standing outside a gay porno
theater in Chicago. "This hippie came walking by and saw me

and recognized me. He stopped and started a conversation. As we talked I could see him registering where I was and his brain was scrambling to comprehend that Ram Dass, the spiritual teacher, was standing in line at the gay porn theater. In my mind I was trying to decide whether to be honest and go into the theater or to just walk down the street with him to get a cup of coffee. I chose to go into the theater. It took a lot of courage for me to do that. My own guilt and shame were so strong."

In the end, Ram Dass decided that, yes, he was more homosexual than bisexual, but that being gay would never be his central, defining characteristic. "Because I live among so many straight populations, I've started to talk more about being bisexual, being involved with men as well as women. Most of the audiences with whom I do that are people who already love me so much they couldn't care if I turned into a frog. Allen Ginsberg goes and confronts people with his gayness. I don't see any reason to do that—it's not my trip. I never deny it, but I don't push it because it's not part of my active identity."

Sexual promiscuity did not make Richard Alpert happy. Later, sexual renunciation did little to foster the spiritual growth of Ram Dass. It only made him "a horny celibate."

"In a still later stage," he explained, "you realize that the aversion is keeping you from being free—and you want to be free, not just high. So you start to come back into who you are, passionate and nonattached. You are fully in life, joyfully participating—sex is a celebration. It's all wonderful, and at the same moment, it's all empty. That's a very evolved stage of spiritual maturation."

Much later in his life, sitting in his home in Hawaii, Ram Dass looks back and sees three great loves in his life—one straight, one gay, and one spiritual. There was Caroline Winter, the girl he met that night back in the sixties at that Grateful Dead concert in San Francisco, the only girl he ever took back to meet his mother. Then there's Peter, a longtime male partner. "I can say to Peter, 'God, I love you so much,' but it's not really a sexual thing. It's been changing. The love goes out and out and out and out. Peter has gone from being a sexual object to my dear friend who I love. He is a person who, from my point of view, goes into the woodwork. The only person now like that is Maharaji. He's my real love. That's just the way it is."

Now, more than ten years after the stroke, Ram Dass has settled down—for the last time, he says—into this spectacular house above the cliffs on the northeast coast of Maui, on the road to Hana. A wealthy benefactor bought the place and rents it to him to use until he dies. There are people here to take care of him. He says he's come here to die, and anyone who wants to see him must now come to Maui. He's done with all that flying around the world, working his wisdom on the consciousness-raising circuit.

Maybe the stroke *was* the best thing to happen to him.

Yet something still shifts in Ram Dass whenever Andrew Weil pops into the story. He's still mad about the way Weil went to Ronnie Winston's father and told him his son had to report Professor Alpert to the Harvard administration, to admit that he gave him drugs. The edge comes back when he talks about the time he met with Weil in the 1970s. Andy had been trying to arrange a meeting to reconcile with the Harvard professor he once brought down. It was the early seventies. Richard Alpert had become Ram Dass. Weil was just making his name as a sympathetic authority on the burgeoning youth drug culture. Ram Dass had finally agreed to meet with his old nemesis. Weil picked him up in his car. Weil remembers taking Ram Dass to the airport. Ram Dass doesn't remember the airport part, but he does remember having a conversation in a car.

"Andrew said to me, 'We turned on the society,'" Ram Dass recalls, barely concealing his condescension. "I remember that the steering wheel was pushing into his stomach. Then he says to me, 'I want to be your student.' I said, 'OK. Lose some weight.' He didn't like that."

Ram Dass laughed. Then shook his head. He wished he hadn't said what he just said. "I know he's done a lot of good work, but

I've had it in my head for so long that he's a bad guy. The way he went after Ronnie's father, that was just . . ."

He didn't finish the sentence, but he didn't have to. It was clear that there was still some reconciliation to be done between Ram Dass and Andrew Weil.

Ram Dass had been sitting in the chair by his picture window for a couple of hours when Andy Weil came up again.

"You know," he said, "I'm sorry about the way I badmouthed . . . what's-his-name."

"You were just being honest."

"Yes," Ram Dass said, paused for a long time, then added, "I was."

"Andy has the impression that you never forgave him."

"You can see that's true," Ram Dass replied. "I should be able to let that go. I should . . ."

Then he leaned back in his orange La-Z-Boy recliner, looked out the picture window at the waves crashing onto the shores of Maui, and sighed a deep sigh.

Trickster
Los Angeles
March 1996

---

They say the best way to predict how a man will handle his death is to look at the way he lived his life. That may or may not be true, but it was certainly the case for Timothy Leary. He lived the life of a showman, a rascal, and a rebel. For Leary, life was a party. Why should death be any different?

Sometime in January 1995, Leary was diagnosed with inoperable prostate cancer. He did not go quietly into the night. He would die in his bed at his home in Los Angeles shortly after midnight on May 31, 1996, ending a sixteen-month media circus in which he floated various stories about how he would turn on, tune in, and drop out one last time. In the mid-1990s, the Internet was the next

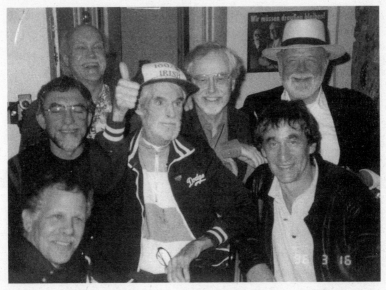

*At a reunion in 1996, just a few weeks before his death, Timothy Leary, with thumb up, is joined (top row, left to right) by Ram Dass, Ralph Metzner, and Paul Lee. Also pictured are three other men who worked with Leary as graduate students at Harvard in the early 1960s—George Litwin, Michael Katz, and Gunter Weil. (Photo courtesy of Paul Lee.)*

big thing. Leary was always fascinated with the next big thing. Cyberspace was the new LSD. Virtual reality was the new reality. Leary would die—*live!*—on the Internet. In the end, he didn't do it, but he livened up his convalescence, and got media attention, by posting his daily drug intake on the Internet. Two cups of caffeine, thirteen cigarettes, two Vicodin, one cocktail, one glass of white wine, one line of cocaine, twelve balloons of nitrous oxide, and Leary Biscuits—marijuana in melted cheese on a Ritz cracker.

Then there was the cryonics scenario. Leary would be frozen until medical science could bring him back. No, just his head would be frozen, kept in the freezer until it could be attached to the body of a beautiful black woman.

Various delegations came to pay their last respects. Six guys who were there when it all began—Richard Alpert, Paul Lee, Ralph Metzner, and three other graduate students who started the

Harvard Psilocybin Project in the fall of 1960—gathered around the dying Leary on March 16, 1996. The high priest of LSD, gaunt with bruised skin and wide eyes receding into his pale face, sat in his wheelchair wearing a blue Dodgers jacket and a baseball cap declaring himself "100% Irish." It was a party, a predeath wake. Leary had surrounded himself with an unruly tribe of young groupies. There was lots of laughter, and smiles all around, but some of Tim's old friends saw beyond the celebration.

Ram Dass, who spent decades working with the sick and dying, saw a lot of denial amid all the partying: "Tim wanted so much to avoid thoughts of death that he tried to keep his life going permanently. All that stuff about freezing his brain. Mostly it was all show biz. But he *was* denying death. I tried to talk to him about it, but I couldn't break through. I worked with his caretakers. I told them how important it was that they try to see his soul, not just the surface Timothy Leary."

Since their breakup back in the mid-1960s, Ram Dass had been watching the Timothy Leary show, mostly from afar. Leary was kicked out of Switzerland in January 1973 and, after a brief stop in Beirut, landed in Kabul, Afghanistan, where he was kidnapped by agents of the U.S. government and brought back to California. In April, he was sentenced to thirty-five years in Folsom State Prison for three prior drug convictions and his 1970 escape from the California Men's Colony in San Luis Obispo. His last year in exile had been consumed by an orgy of constant drug use—marijuana, Quaaludes, cocaine, heroin, and a mind-warping marathon of LSD intoxication. It's not surprising that large sections of his much-anticipated account of those years, the Bantam paperback titled *Confessions of a Hope Fiend,* were a jumble of incomprehensible fantasies.

Leary's latest consort, Joanna Harcourt-Smith, tried to keep the convict in the public eye and his appeal hopes alive with a series of benefits and press conferences. "His mind is already freed," she said. "All we need now is his body."

Leary's actions and bizarre writings made it seem like the man had lost his mind. Such a conclusion seemed to be warranted considering the mountain of mind-altering drugs he'd taken. But Leary's brain was still in fine shape. At his March 1973 trial, a criminal psychologist testified that Leary had just scored "genius level" on a standardized intelligence test. He was also given the standardized creativity test and got the highest score the psychologist had ever witnessed.

Leary would soon show the world that he was smart enough to talk his way out of prison, and he would do so by ratting on his friends, including several lawyers who were alleged intermediaries in the Weather Underground caper to smuggle Leary out of the country and into Algeria. Working in collusion with Joanna Harcourt-Smith and the FBI, Leary turned over boxes of documents from his archives while Harcourt-Smith wore a wire in an effort to entrap several associates who helped Leary and his previous wife, Rosemary, elude the FBI and make their way to Algeria.

As part of his deal with the government, Leary even tried—unsuccessfully—to get Rosemary to come out of hiding and join him as a federal informant. In a handwritten letter penned at the FBI offices in southern California on June 1, 1974, Leary portrayed himself as a loyal, law-abiding citizen of the United States of America. "It was a mistake in judgment for us to get involved with dope dealers and illegal revolutionaries," he wrote. "Please do not fear the American law or American law enforcement officials. . . . The old polarities and conflicts of the sixties are over."


Word soon got out that the high priest of LSD had become a government snitch. A group of Leary associates—including Jerry Rubin, Allen Ginsberg, and Ram Dass—convened a press conference in San Francisco to denounce their old friend. Leary's twenty-four-year-old son, Jack, joined the proceedings and condemned his father. "Timothy Leary lies at will when he thinks it will benefit him," his son said. "He finds lies easier to control than the truth. And he creates fantastic absurd stories which he gets caught up in, and then cannot distinguish them from the truth."

One longtime Leary associate, Gene Schoenfeld, could not believe that his old friend had become a government snitch. Schoenfeld, better known at the time as Dr. Hip, had a medical-advice program on alternative radio stations and an underground-newspaper column. Schoenfeld had also been the Leary family doctor when Tim, Rosemary, Jack, and Susan were all living in Berkeley in the late 1960s. He didn't believe the story that Leary had turned against his old friends. He also didn't think it was right that the organizers of the press conference had brought Jack Leary into the proceedings to denounce his famous father.

Dr. Hip decided the press conference was a kangaroo court. To make his point, in true sixties style, he obtained a kangaroo suit from a friend who ran a costume shop. Schoenfeld climbed into the suit, grabbed a coconut cream pie, and hopped into the press conference at the St. Francis Hotel. His plan was to throw the pie in Jerry Rubin's face. "I had these boxing gloves on so I wasn't able to get the Saran Wrap off the pie. Then someone started pulling me off the stage, and in the process, pulled my head off. There was a gasp in the audience when people saw it was me."

Schoenfeld was later shown a grand jury transcript that convinced him that both Tim and Joanna Harcourt-Smith, who became Leary's partner following the breakup of his fourth marriage, had, in fact, been government informants.

Dr. Hip knew that the prison time was getting to Leary. He'd visited him a few times and saw that his confinement, coming on top of nearly two decades of weekly LSD trips, was finally taking a toll on the mind of Timothy Leary. Tim was convinced he'd be locked up for the rest of his life, and he would do anything to get out. "One time when I visited him in prison he accused me of having an affair with Joanna. Then he said something about how he could summon up evil forces from the earth and direct them at me. I thought, 'This is not a good sign.'"

That wasn't the first time Schoenfeld wondered about Leary's sanity: "When he was running for governor of California, he actually started believing that he might win. Tim was very charismatic, but he was a bit of a megalomaniac. I remember back in the sixties there were all these psychedelic posters that portrayed Tim as some kind of God. Tim liked that kind of adulation. At a certain point, he became the victim of his own image."

It would take two years, but in April 1976 Leary finally walked out of jail and into the Federal Witness Protection Program. Within a few months, he was scheduling a new round of media interviews, starting with a spread in *People* magazine. Over the next two decades, there would be various crusades—starting with space migration—and assorted attempts to make a comeback. Most of his friends eventually forgave him for his indiscretions with the FBI. In 1983, Leary and Ram Dass shared a stage at Harvard to celebrate the twentieth anniversary of their expulsion from the ivy-covered halls. Seven years later, they were at the podium at the Claremont Hotel in Berkeley, where they and six hundred other proponents of enlightenment through modern chemistry came together for a discussion titled "Psychedelics in the 1990s: Regulation or Prohibition." Ram Dass thought back to the early sixties and had to laugh at their naiveté. "Tim and I actually had a chart on the wall about how soon everyone would be enlightened," he said. "We found out that real change is harder. We downplayed the fact that the psychedelic experience isn't for everyone."


Seven years later, Leary was lying on his deathbed, surrounded by a new generation of devotees. One of them, Robert Forte, was just a young kid in the 1960s. Forte hadn't really thought much about the life and times of Timothy Leary until the late 1970s, when he was a student at the University of California at Santa Cruz. His introduction to Leary came through Frank Barron, the man who first opened Leary's eyes to the wonders of magic mushrooms. Barron, who'd studied with Leary at Berkeley in the 1950s, had moved to Santa Cruz in 1969, where he taught a popular course at the University of California campus there on the psychology of creativity.

Forte became interested in the expanding field of consciousness research. He met Leary in the 1980s, but he didn't really get to know the man until the 1990s. His fascination with the sixties icon deepened in 1993, when Forte attended an LSD conference in Switzerland. The assembly had been convened by Sandoz Pharmaceuticals Company and the Swiss Academy of Medicine to mark the fiftieth anniversary of the drug's discovery by Sandoz chemist Albert Hofmann. It was mainly a gathering of psychiatric researchers, and most of them mentioned Leary's name with a dismissive and scornful tone. They blamed Leary's messianic crusade for the subsequent crackdown on serious research into the properties and potentialities of LSD.

People love to blame Timothy Leary for all the casualties of the sixties drug culture—for all those people who suffered serious mental problems after taking LSD or who later became addicted to other drugs. Gather together a large group of people from that era and you're likely to find someone who will blame Timothy Leary for the suicide of a friend or loved one. Some of this criticism is unfair. Leary and Alpert, at least in their early years at Harvard and Millbrook, always stressed that LSD should be taken in a safe setting by someone ready to deal with whatever psychological and emotional issues were likely to arise. They were the cautious advocates of psychedelic drug exploration—especially when compared with the scene out on the West Coast, where Ken Kesey and his Merry Pranksters were indiscriminately dosing the crowds at rock concerts and "Acid Tests." At the same time, it was Leary's own proselytizing that made him the lightning rod for critics of sixties excess. Leary loved to take the credit—but not the blame—for the drug revolution of the 1960s and '70s. "Seven million people I turned on," he said near the end of his life, "and only one hundred thousand have come by to thank me."

Forte lived at the house on Sunbrook Drive during the last few weeks of Leary's life. He accompanied Leary's son, Jack, on a flight from San Francisco to Los Angeles. They had been estranged since the 1970s. Leary's other child, his daughter, Susan, suffered from severe psychological problems during much of her life, and committed suicide in 1990. Jack Leary hadn't seen his father since they crossed paths at a private memorial service that had been held for his sister. On the flight down to L.A., Forte was amazed at how much Jack looked like early photos of Leary when he was teaching at Harvard. Forte was trying to prepare Jack for the deathbed meeting with his estranged father.

"What was remarkable to me was his lack of affect, how he was so cool—just an ordinary guy getting on a plane," Forte recalled. "I said, 'Wow, when I don't see my dad for a year or so I'm all nervous and here you haven't seen your father for fifteen years. You seem remarkably calm.'"

"He wasn't really a father to me," Jack replied.

Paul Lee, the Harvard Divinity School graduate who worked with Leary in the early years, paid for Jack Leary's plane ticket and was there when father met son. "We were hoping that they would reconcile, or that Jack would at least show up," Lee said. "I'm not sure it really worked. It was pretty frigid. Tim was pleased to see him, but Jack was real stiff."

In the end, Timothy Leary kicked the cryonics crowd out of his house. His body was cremated, but he would have one last posthumous blast. Almost a year after he died, a small glass vial containing some of his ashes was blasted into outer space aboard a Pegasus rocket launched from the Canary Islands. Twenty-five people had prepaid a private company to send their remains into orbit. Joining Leary on the flight was a little bit of Gene Roddenberry, the man who created *Star Trek.*

Forte spent the last few weeks of Leary's life trying to figure out what this man was all about. "Was Tim a wise man or was he a psychopathic egotistical maniac, or both?" Forte asked himself. "I'd hang out with him until three in the morning. Sometimes he would appear like a nonordinary being. There was a tangible aura. He would glow. Sometimes he was just so clear and present and positive, but other times he would just morph into this twisted, angry, fucked-up old man."

Leary was different things to different people. He was reviled. He was revered. He was a prophet. He was a phony. He was a brilliant, innovative thinker. He was a fool. He captured the irreverent, rebellious spirit of the sixties. He was a fame-seeking, manipulative con artist. Who was he? Perhaps The Trickster said it best when he quipped, "You get the Timothy Leary you deserve."

## Teacher
## San Diego
## November 2007

Friends and fans of Huston Smith were gathered at a San Diego restaurant to honor the man and celebrate the fiftieth anniversary of the publication of his landmark book, originally titled *The Religions of Man.* The event was held in conjunction with the annual meeting of the American Academy of Religion, which draws tens of thousands of scholars, graduate students, writers, editors, publishers, and others who make a living studying and otherwise explaining the various ways people approach God and try to understand the meaning of it all. Huston had not been feeling well in recent months. There were problems with his hip and problems with his hearing and all those other maladies that beset a man approaching his ninetieth birthday. Huston came late to the party, hobbling in with the assistance of a friend and a walker. He was barely noticed by most of the crowd, who were busy enjoying the open bar and luscious hors d'oeuvres.

His publisher made the introduction, mentioning that more than two million copies of the book have been sold over the last five decades. The book continues to sell about four thousand copies a month. The publisher told a story about running into an older woman and her grown daughter standing in line at one of Huston's book signings. She had come to thank Huston. She'd read his book, now titled *The World's Religions,* decades ago. It had transformed the way she looked at matters of faith. The woman's daughter had recently come home from college and couldn't stop talking about this book she'd been assigned in one of her classes, a book titled *The World's Religions.*

Professor Smith was handed the microphone. His voice was shaky, but his spirit shone through. He didn't say much, but what he said left tears in more than a few eyes.

Huston began by pulling an old letter from his pocket. A respected religion scholar had written it to him nearly fifty years ago. The woman who wrote the letter was long dead, but her words came down like a voice from heaven.

"Dear Huston," the letter read, "I have spent the afternoon reading your book. I read it all the way through and then I sat down and read it all the way through again. . . . I want you to know that when you are an old man you will look back on the young man who wrote this book with a great deal of love and affection."

Huston is not alone. If the measure of a man's life is the number of people who remember him with love and affection, Huston Smith measures up. All four members of the Harvard Psychedelic Club dedicated their lives to the study of the human consciousness, including chemically induced altered states of consciousness. What separates Huston and Ram Dass is their understanding that the real test of a person's spirit is the way they live their lives. It's what happens *after* the ecstasy.

Smith has lived a full life, personally and professionally. In 2009, he celebrated both his ninetieth birthday and his sixty-sixth wedding anniversary with Kendra. Huston knew she was the one from the beginning. He had dated other young women, but there was something different about the daughter of theologian H. N. Wieman. Their date ended with a political debate. Kendra was totally behind Norman Thomas, the Socialist candidate for president in 1940. Huston wasn't so sure. "There was none of the usual gazing deep into my eyes and nodding agreement with everything I said," he recalled decades later. "Her physical charms are noteworthy, but what I find distinctive is her mind. She has ideas, stands up for them, and is articulate and persuasive." Their marriage produced three daughters, Karen, Gael, and Kimberly, but Kendra was more than just a wife and mother. She was a lifelong partner in Huston's work. She was there in Timothy Leary's house on New Year's Day, 1961, taking a stronger dose of psychedelics than Huston dared to swallow.

In 1957, just two years after the publication of *The Religions of Man,* Kendra accompanied Huston on a months-long round-the-world pilgrimage. The trip was paid for by William H. Danforth, who'd made a fortune selling animal feed with the Ralston Purina Company. The businessman had seen Huston lecturing on the world's religions in a series of programs Smith hosted in the early days of public television. "I understand that some of the religions you are teaching in your television course are in countries you have not been to," Danforth wrote. "If the university would grant you a semester's leave and you added your summer vacation to it, a check to fund a round-the-world trip for you and your wife will be in the return mail." The trip took Huston and Kendra from the Cathedral of Notre Dame in Paris to the Lascaux cave paintings in the south of France; from Vatican City, where Huston had his wallet lifted at a high pontifical mass, to Athens and Jerusalem; from Istanbul, where they were entranced by the Muslim call to prayer, to Tehran, where they watched the whirling dervishes; and on to Burma, India, and Japan. It was the first of many international sojourns Huston would take over his long life, including a meeting with the Dalai Lama in Dharamsala, an encounter with aborigines in Australia, and a memorable trek through the African bush. Closer to home, when he was a graduate student at Berkeley in the 1940s, Huston hopped over to San Francisco to witness the founding of the United Nations. In 1989, he just happened to find himself in Beijing when the Chinese student uprising broke out in Tiananmen Square. He sat down in interviews and other encounters with a string of noteworthy Americans, including Eleanor Roosevelt, theologian Reinhold Niebuhr, and the Reverend Martin

Luther King Jr. For years, Huston resisted efforts to get him to write a personal memoir of his long and eventful life. He was more interested in the human search for meaning than he was in one man's story, even if that story was his own. But in the spring of 2009, in his ninetieth year, Huston finally relented, and his publisher released an autobiography, *Tales of Wonder: Adventures Chasing the Divine.*

As he entered his ninth decade, Huston Smith had buried his parents and one of his daughters, and lived through the bizarre disappearance and presumed death of one of his granddaughters. His father, the man who went to China to "Christianize the world," died at Ozarks Methodist Manor, a retirement community south of Springfield, Missouri. Huston and Kendra's oldest daughter, Karen, died of cancer when she was just fifty years old. As she awaited her death, Karen threw a party to celebrate her father's seventy-fifth birthday. Karen had converted to Judaism when she married, and in her last sustained conversation with her father, she spoke of angels. "I sensed at once," Huston says, "that she was thinking of the Kabalistic view in which every mitzvah (good deed) that people perform creates an angel. Those angels don't vanish with the acts that brought them into being. They live on as permanent additions to the universe, affecting the balance between the forces of good and evil." Then, in 2002, one of Huston's grandchildren, Serena, disappeared under suspicious circumstances and was presumed dead after she vanished from a boat sailing in the South Pacific. She had been sailing with her boyfriend, Bison Dele, an NBA star who had suddenly given up a promising career in professional basketball and headed off to Tahiti. Authorities believe Dele's troubled brother murdered him and Serena, but their bodies were never found.

Death is the final act of every life, but for the person of faith, it is more like an intermission between this life and the next. Every world religion has its vision of the afterlife. One reason Smith was so drawn to Hinduism was its doctrine of universal salvation. Those who believe in reincarnation hold that the soul comes back to earth

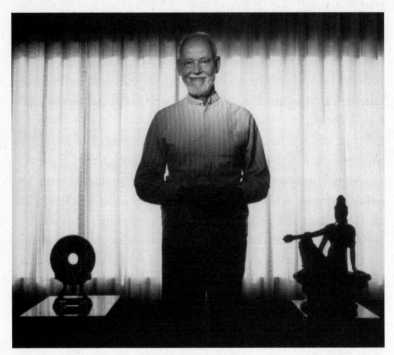

*Huston Smith (Photo by Anne Hamersky.)*

to take care of any unfinished business. How many times we return depends on the way we live our lives, but in the end, everyone is saved. Huston Smith never renounced the faith of his forefathers, but he always had a problem with the whole idea of eternal damnation. Smith believes in religious tolerance and mutual respect as much as he believes in God. And he had always struggled to reconcile that belief with the idea of sinners and nonbelievers burning in hell for all eternity.

For much of his life, Huston fought that monstrous doctrine. Then, one day in 1964, he found himself in the foothills of the Himalayas. He was on sabbatical from the university and off interviewing a number of gurus, trying to deepen his knowledge of the religions of India. That's when Huston stumbled across a mysterious figure that would help him gain new understanding of his own Christian faith. His name was Father Lazarus, and he was a missionary with the Eastern Orthodox Church. He appeared one day in the doorway of a bungalow in the Himalayas, tall, dressed in white, and sporting a full beard. He'd spent the last twenty years in India.

Huston and Father Lazarus spent a week tramping around the Himalayan foothills, talking nonstop about the church, the Bible, and other matters of faith. Huston shared his revulsion with the doctrine of eternal damnation, and the priest suggested that he take another look at a passage in Second Corinthians, where Saint Paul tells the story of a man caught up in the third heaven. What struck Father Lazarus about the story is the way Paul repeats a mysterious aspect of the man's story. "Whether in the body or out of it," Paul says, "I do not know." The great apostle goes on to explain that, in heaven, the man in question "heard things that were not to be told, that no mortal is permitted to repeat." Father Lazarus was convinced that the secret of which Paul spoke is that there is a third heaven in which *everyone* is saved.

That conversation stuck with Huston Smith, and helped him come to terms with his own passing. "After I shed my body, I will continue to be conscious of the life I have lived and the people who remain on earth. Sooner or later, however, there will come a time when no one alive will have heard of Huston Smith, let alone have known him, whereupon there ceases to be any point in my hanging around." During his life Huston came to believe that people turn to religion the way sunflowers bend in the direction of the light. We reach for God "in the way that the wings of birds point to the reality of air." Someday, Huston believes, he will turn his back on planet earth and set his gaze upon the beatific vision. Mystic by temperament, if not attainment, Huston will enjoy that sunset. Toward the end, he expects to "oscillate back and forth between enjoying the sunset and enjoying Huston-Smith-enjoying-the-sunset."

In the end, Huston expects to find the uncompromised sunset more absorbing. "The string will have been cut," he says. "The bird will be free."

# Healer, Teacher, Trickster, Seeker

Fourteen years before Timothy Leary and Richard Alpert were kicked out of Harvard, another pair of Boston drug researchers conducted their own experiments on a group of undergraduate students. History has all but forgotten Dr. Max Rinkel and Dr. Robert Hyde. But their story is worth telling, if only because it provides a larger context to understand the events of this book.

Rinkel and Hyde were using a new drug called LSD-25, which was many times stronger than the magic mushroom pills later employed by the Harvard Psilocybin Project. But the most important difference between these two research projects was the motivation behind the experiments. Both projects were playing with the minds of young Harvard students, but they came at their work with very different expectations. Leary and Alpert hoped to show that their subjects could experience joyous moments of mystical insight. Rinkel and Hyde were trying to discover how LSD could drive their subjects crazy, how it could provoke a "transitory psychotic disturbance."

Is this simply two ways of describing the same thing? Perhaps. But the intent of the researcher is important. And that is especially true for psychedelic researchers, whose expectations and intent almost certainly influence the outcome of their experiments.

Historians of the psychedelic era tell us that the first LSD trip in North America was most likely the initial trip taken by Dr. Robert Hyde. It happened sometime in early 1949, just six years after the Swiss chemist Albert Hofmann discovered the powerful effects triggered by LSD. Rinkel and Hyde conducted their experiments on about a hundred students at the Boston Psychopathic Institute, a mental-health clinic affiliated with Harvard University. They reported their findings at the May 1950 meeting of the American Psychiatric Association. Yes, they concluded, LSD could easily be used to provoke temporary psychosis.

One would think that would have been the end of their research. After all, who would want to intentionally drive research subjects crazy? What's the social benefit behind such a twisted research agenda?

It would be decades before we would learn the answer to those questions. The explanation would come only when it was revealed that Rinkel and Hyde's research was secretly funded by the Central Intelligence Agency. Their experiments were part of a vast government program in the 1950s to see if LSD could be used for military purposes as a chemical warfare agent. Perhaps it could be sprayed on enemy troops—a powerful weapon of mass *distraction*. Maybe it could be employed as a truth serum for interrogating prisoners of war. Then there was the idea that enemy soldiers could be drugged, hypnotized, and programmed to go back behind enemy lines and sabotage their comrades in arms.

Philip Slater, one of the Harvard graduate students who administered LSD under the supervision of Dr. Hyde, had no idea that two CIA front groups were funding their research. Slater was twenty-five years old when he signed on to assist Robert Hyde, but he didn't find out about the CIA connections until sometime in the 1980s, when Slater was in his sixties. Slater worked on the project from 1952 to 1954. He estimates that about half of the subjects were undergraduates. He doesn't recall exactly what the students were told they would be given, but he believes they knew it would somehow affect their mental processes. At the time, the word *psychedelic* had not been coined, and the Cambridge researchers classified LSD as a "psychotomimetic" drug, meaning that it mimicked psychosis. Their job was to find out exactly what kind of psychosis the drug induced. Student volunteers were dosed individually and in groups. About three hours after they took the drug, when they were at the peak of their experience, they would be sent down to the hospital's admitting psychiatrist for diagnosis. Such categories as schizophrenic, paranoid, and manic-depressive were used to describe their condition.

Not surprisingly, some of the subjects were deeply disturbed by all this. "We lost a couple," Slater recalled. "One had to be hospitalized. Another went out in the street to see if cars were real. That really scared us."

Hardly anyone had heard of LSD in the early 1950s. Aldous Huxley had yet to take his first mescaline trip and write *The Doors of Perception*. R. Gordon Wasson had not yet returned from Mexico to sing the praises of magic mushrooms in the pages of *Life* magazine. If Slater, Rinkel, and Hyde had any preconceptions about LSD—ideas that would affect the actual experience of taking the drug—their expectations were that their subjects would go through a period of temporary psychosis.

Slater initially saw LSD as a test of his sanity, so when he resisted the experience, he found that it produced relatively mild effects. There were no hallucinations. But then he and other friends started sneaking doses out of the hospital. They began taking the drug in less formal settings. They began to see something else. "All you had to do was walk off and look at a plant and you'd start having all these visual changes," he said. "It definitely felt like we were expanding our consciousness. From that moment, we saw the world differently than people who had not had the experience."

Like Timothy Leary, Slater couldn't take the academic world all that seriously after his psychedelic experience. He taught sociology at Harvard and Brandeis. He played the game for fifteen years. He went out to the West Coast for a teaching job at the newly established University of California at Santa Cruz, but he knew that his taking the post was just an excuse to get away and change his life. Slater taught at Santa Cruz for only a couple of years. Like Leary, he'd seen the absurdity of academic pretension. Then, in 1971, his book *The Pursuit of Loneliness: American Culture at the Breaking Point* became a surprise bestseller.

Decades later, I made an appointment to meet Phil Slater at a coffee house in Santa Cruz. I was sitting outside when a guy pulled up on a bicycle. Could that be him?

Slater had to be well into his eighties. This trim man with a full head of gray hair looked to be in his late fifties or early sixties. It *was* Slater. At the time, I was still interviewing people for this book, and just starting to figure out what it all might mean. Something told me this psychedelic pioneer, this rebel sociologist, could point me in the right direction.

"What Leary did more than anything else was activate conservative anxiety in America," Slater said. "The way he phrased the rejection of the status quo fit the hippies and the political left, and he did it in a way that scared people hugely. While all the hippies and feminists and the radicals and the civil rights people argued about which was the most important way to go, the only people who really understood that it was all one thing was the right wing."

That's most certainly true. Timothy Leary helped provoke the "war on drugs" and Richard Nixon's larger campaign against the sixties counterculture and the New Left. He was also a factor in the rise of Ronald Reagan and the conservative backlash of the 1980s. After all, Timothy Leary was the acid trickster, the joker who danced around Reagan's earlier campaign to become governor of California. But Leary did something else. There was more to all this than simply the backlash against it.

"Leary was the mouth," Slater said. "He gave voice to something people were feeling privately. 'Oh, this is not just me. This is not just *my* experience. This is reality. This is essential reality.'"

There's the key, the Rosetta stone that brings together the work of the Harvard Psychedelic Club. Timothy Leary, Richard Alpert, Andrew Weil, and Huston Smith did nothing less than inspire a generation of Americans to redefine the nature of reality. People who have taken LSD or other psychedelic drugs see the world differently than those who have not. But the story does not stop there.

The psychedelic experience is a powerful experience, but it does not end with the experience. What happens next? How do we live our lives? What happens after the ecstasy? We see the world in a different way, but what do we do with that realization?

None of the men of the Harvard Psychedelic Club officially fall into that demographic leviathan known as "the baby boomers," but the generation born in the aftermath of World War II *was* their primary audience. Many of these kids were Spock babies, so-called because they were raised by parents taking the advice of Dr. Benjamin Spock, the influential American pediatrician. His main message was that children need to think that anything is possible. Those of us boomers who grew into counterculturists or revolutionaries tried to live out that prescription, and many of us turned for a time to psychedelic drugs to broaden our vision of what was possible. We did not always live out our visions, but at least we sought them out. Perhaps the historical importance of Leary, Alpert, Weil, and Smith is not so much any particular vision, but the very process of envisioning. For a moment in time, we had the experience of expanding our minds, and one of the side effects of that condition is envisioning an alternative way to live.

Leary was The Trickster; his rebel spirit provided the signal to those of us who chose to listen. It was time to move beyond the limited vision of the 1950s, time to search for something new, even if we weren't sure *what* it was. Alpert was The Seeker. He took the search to the Far East and brought it back for those of us who couldn't go there in body but longed to be there in spirit. Smith was The Teacher, continuing the journey to all the religions of the world, showing us that in the most basic way, the spirit remains the same. He moved us beyond the drug experience into a deeper understanding of the mystical experience as something that should bring us together, not drive us apart. In the end, Weil became The Healer. He worked to bring the psychedelic vision down to earth, to more fully understand the connection between the body and the mind and, through that understanding, change the way we look at sickness and disease, health and well-being.

That's all true, but there's another side to the story of the psychedelic sixties. We shouldn't get too swept away in all the oneness and the wonder and the healing. Let's not forget the many lives that were lost along the way. Many of us took the potion but never found the cure. We see those damaged children of the sixties in the life of Hunter Thompson, the gonzo journalist who consumed at least as much LSD as Timothy Leary. Hunter never seemed to get beyond the bemused cynicism that limited so many of us. "What Leary took down with him," Hunter wrote, "was the central illusion of a whole lifestyle that he helped to create—a generation of permanent cripples and failed seekers who never understood the essential old mystic fallacy of the acid culture, the desperate assumption that somebody or at least some force was tending the light at the end of the tunnel."

There's some hard truth in Hunter's words, but they come from a tortured soul who blew his mind out with drugs before blowing his brains out with a handgun. Hunter was right, up to a point. Many people *were* crippled by the acid culture, but many more were not. It's easy to parody the spiritual seekers who flocked to India in the 1960s and 1970s, but many of them returned with the central truth that helped them live better lives.

Many of us danced with the angels of the drug culture, only to be brought down by the demon of addiction. There *was* a serious problem of drug abuse in this country in the 1960s and the 1970s. There was also a serious problem of drug abuse in this country in the 1950s and the 1980s, especially if one includes alcoholic beverages in the category of "recreational drugs." The only thing that changes is which drugs are licit and which drugs are illicit, which ones doctors prescribe, which ones are sold at your local supermarket, and which ones are peddled on the street.

If we can believe the various surveys of drug use in America, the percentage of young people taking LSD increased until the mid-

1970s. Those numbers declined in the 1980s, but were back to 1975 levels by the mid-1990s. Then LSD use sharply declined in the first decade of the twenty-first century. Experts disagree over the reasons behind the sudden drop-off in recent years, but it appears to have been caused by an interruption in the supply of ingredients needed to produce LSD, along with the rise of other drugs, such as Ecstasy (MDMA) and salvia divinorum, a powerful psychedelic plant that was legal and easy to obtain over the Internet. Another clear trend over the last twenty years has been an increase in the recreational use and abuse of drugs manufactured by pharmaceutical companies—especially downers like OxyContin and Vicodin, and uppers like Ritalin and Adderall.

America has been calling for temperance or declaring war on (some) drugs since 1785, when Dr. Benjamin Rush, one of the signers of the Declaration of Independence, wrote an anti-liquor tract titled *An Inquiry into the Effects of Ardent Spirits upon the Human Body and Mind*. Over the last century, Prohibition came and went. Cocaine was touted as a wonder drug, an invigorating tonic, a relatively harmless party drug, and a poison responsible for the breakdown of the African-American communities across the nation.

Timothy Leary did not inspire the war on drugs all by himself. Yet he *was* largely to blame for the crackdown on responsible psychedelic drug research in the United States. Leary rarely pops up in the headlines anymore, but he did in the spring of 2007, when *Time* magazine asked the question "Was Timothy Leary Right?" The article discusses how—for the first time since Leary and Alpert were disciplined in 1963—both Harvard and the National Institute of Mental Health were doing research into the therapeutic use of Ecstasy. That's the drug that fueled all those late-night raves way back in the 1990s. *Time* also reports in that story that a British foundation had just gotten government approval to begin the first human studies with LSD since the 1970s.

Leary remained a dropout, but Huston Smith, Richard Alpert, and Andrew Weil each found their way back into mainstream culture and helped transform it. Weil abandoned his plans for a career in the medical establishment, but only to take a more holistic approach to health care. Smith saw the hedonism of the drug movement and the messianic complex of its leader. He cut his ties to Leary and went back to the classroom. Alpert abandoned his career as a university research psychologist and became a spiritual teacher. None of them followed Leary's advice. They turned on, tuned in, but they did not drop out—at least not permanently.

All four of these characters played a role in the social and spiritual changes that made the sixties such a pivotal decade in recent American history. They stirred up the water and then rode a wave of social change. The difference is that Timothy Leary never found an anchor, the stability needed to bring those changes into his life in a positive, long-lasting way. Instead of finding an anchor, Leary tried to walk on the water.

Perhaps it's not surprising that Andrew Weil, the youngest and most ambitious member of the Harvard Psychedelic Club, had the greatest long-term impact on American culture. Weil's main contribution has been his work on the much-needed reformation of the American health-care system. He has led the crusade for what he calls integrative medicine, which takes the best from East and West, combining Western medical technology with meditation and healing practices involving diet, yoga, and acupuncture. His Center for Integrative Medicine at the University of Arizona has been instrumental in setting up similar programs at medical centers across the United States. His work has inspired medical practitioners to prescribe meditation and other relaxation techniques to lower stress, reduce the risk of heart disease, and strengthen the immune system—one of the clearest examples of how a counterculture practice has mainstreamed into American life.

Richard Alpert, as Ram Dass, inspired the thrill seekers of my generation to go beyond the revelatory insights that psychedelic drugs provide and pursue a less dangerous, and more life-affirming, spiritual practice. Ram Dass helped popularize the meditation techniques now used in Weil's East-meets-West medical programs. Alpert was a trailblazer, and the counterculture's most articulate and accessible tour guide, especially for those of us trying to come down off the acid and learn something from the experience, such as how to live our lives with more consciousness and compassion.

Huston Smith's impact has been subtler, but significant. Recent surveys of the American religious landscape show that while religious belief is relatively stable, religious affiliation is in decline. One of the fastest-growing religious groups in the United States is the "nones," as in "none of the above." These are people who say "none" when pollsters ask them their religious affiliation. Some "nones" identify themselves as atheists or agnostics, but the vast majority believe in God. They pray and/or meditate. Many describe themselves as "spiritual but not religious." These surveys also show rising religious tolerance—among both the affiliated and the unaffiliated. There are many factors behind these trends, but one of them is certainly the life work of Huston Smith.

In the two years since I began working on this book, there have been a few changes in the lives of the surviving members of the Harvard Psychedelic Club. Huston Smith moved out of his Berkeley home and into an assisted-living facility. He may be in his nineties, but Huston still finds the energy to give an occasional public talk. Ram Dass fell out of his wheelchair and broke his hip, reducing his already limited mobility. It's been almost two years since he told me that he "came to Maui to die," yet he continues to teach on the Internet and welcomes seekers coming to Hawaii on spiritual retreat.

Leary has been dead more than a decade, but Weil remains a vital force. On a rainy night in 2009, he stood before a sold-out audience of three thousand attentive listeners at the Paramount Theater in Oakland, California, delivering, without notes, an inspiring, informative hourlong lecture, followed by a thirty-minute question-and-answer session. Two weeks later, Weil was in Washington, D.C., to testify before a Senate committee drafting legislation to overhaul the way Americans fund and receive medical care.

Timothy Leary, Huston Smith, Richard Alpert, and Andrew Weil came together in an extraordinary time of social upheaval and unbridled hope—those thousand days between the election and assassination of President John F. Kennedy, a man who seemed to embody the youth and vigor of the next generation. Kennedy was elected in the fall of 1960, the same season during which Andrew Weil and the rest of the class of 1964 came to Harvard to begin their undergraduate studies. It was a time of openness and optimism, and it all seemed to come crashing down on a single day, November 22, 1963. Two things of note happened that day. President Kennedy was assassinated in Dallas, and Aldous Huxley died at his home in Los Angeles. Several hours before Kennedy was shot, Huxley's wife, Laura, sat at his side and administered a dose of LSD to usher the famous writer out of this world and into the next. And it was Timothy Leary who visited Huxley two days before his death, delivering the drugs for that final trip.

The murder of President Kennedy, followed in tragic succession by the assassinations of Robert Kennedy and Martin Luther King Jr., could have killed the sixties, but that era's enlivening spirit somehow survived. Deconstructing a decade is a formidable task. All kinds of forces were at work in the unfolding of the 1960s—the post–World War II economic boom, the civil rights movement, the sexual revolution, the war in Vietnam, feminism, ecological awareness, and the human-potential movement. It was also a time when Americans began to see the limits of U.S. military and economic power and started looking for new ways to be part of an increasingly interconnected world.

Assessing the impact of the psychedelic movement on all this is tricky at best. We have to look deeply, into the DNA of these movements, to see the psychedelic vision at work. In some ways, the impact is obvious. The holistic feeling these drugs unleashed helped millions of us find new ways of looking at our mind, body, and spirit, and, through that new vision, it sparked a movement that would change the way we think about our mental health, our physical well-being, and our spiritual search for a power beyond our skin-encapsulated egotistical selves. The sixties were such a divisive decade that, when we look back on it, we tend to forget that the "counterculture" was not just against everything. The antiwar movement was for peace. The civil rights and feminist movements were for equality. The environmental movement was not just against pollution; it was for a new way of seeing the interdependence of all living things.

Psychedelics inspired many of us to take a more positive, expansive view of our potential as human beings. Psychologists transcended Freud. Sociologists and political scientists moved beyond Marx. Cynics, skeptics, and hard-core materialists suddenly found themselves interested in the spiritual quest. People of faith began to see beyond the doctrines and dogma of their own religious traditions to envision a more inclusive understanding of the contemplative core that runs through all world religions.

We may not like to admit it now, but many of us turned on, tuned in, and dropped out, at least for a while. We saw the light. We began to question the materialist, consumerist mind-set into which we were raised and started looking for other ways to be. We learned to laugh at ourselves, and at much of what was going on around us. Many of us turned our back on that vision in the eighties and the nineties, when corporate America roared back into our lives with a vengeance. Many of us spent decades amassing at least enough material wealth to see the world, raise our families, send our kids to college, and plan for our retirement. But at least we tried to find another way. Now, more than ever, we need to remember the lessons of that idealistic era. It's time, once again, to find new ways to live together with equality, justice, and compassion.

Richard Alpert, Timothy Leary, Huston Smith, and Andrew Weil each laid a cornerstone for what would be built—and what can still be built—from the progressive vision of the psychedelic sixties. The story does not end with them, for the forces they helped unleash were immeasurably larger than those four men, and the changes they wrought are still with us today. They changed the way we view the world, heal ourselves, and practice religion.

They changed the way we see the very nature of reality. We see the best of them in the best of ourselves. In the end, it's not about the drugs. It's about remembering all the life-affirming moments along the way—those glimpses of wonder and awe, empathy and interconnectedness—and finding a place for all of that in the rest of our lives.

# AFTERWORD

This book was not about me, yet I owe it to the reader—and perhaps myself—to end with a personal story, one that helps explain why I spent two years of my life chronicling four other peoples' lives.

It happened at the end of that era we've come to call "the sixties." Julia and I were starting our first year of studies at the University of California at Berkeley. We'd just met, fallen in love, and decided it would be extremely far-out to drive down to Big Sur, drop some acid, and spend the weekend camping on the central California coast. We threw two sleeping bags and ourselves into my red 1965 Mustang, which had a white vinyl roof and two McGovern bumper stickers plastered across the rear window. We arrived sometime in the midafternoon, pulled off Highway One, and parked the car under a small stand of Monterey pines. We looked at each other, smiled, and carefully laid two tiny pieces of LSD-infused blotter paper onto our tongues.

We had just enough time to wander through a maze of scratchy manzanita and down to a stand of whimsical sandstone formations sculpted atop a windswept cliff. There were the usual early warning signs as we started coming onto the acid—a queasy stomach and that uneasy feeling that accompanies the first tugs on the existential anchor. That feeling passed quickly. There was that familiar shift in pattern recognition that often comes with the psychedelic experience, when you suddenly notice the wonderful symmetry of nature and interconnectedness of things that once seemed separate. Colors get brighter; the air seems fresher and more alive. We stopped on a bluff high above the crashing waves and swirling tide pools, where we soon found ourselves too stoned to stand up. We dropped to our knees like we were no longer separate beings, and then rolled over on our sides, unconcerned that we were just a few feet from the edge of the cliff.

We started to melt together. I'd curled up into a fetal position. Julia was tall and thin, more or less equaling my six-foot frame, so she could easily wrap her arms and legs around my torso. At first, it felt like I was inside of her, like an unborn child. Then I was born again. Then we merged together like we were one being—physically, emotionally, intellectually, and spiritually. All we saw was white light, but we somehow continued communicating with each other. Not with words, but through some other means of communion. Time stopped, or at least it slowed down to a glacial pace. Such a feeling of, of, um . . . *suchness*.

Neither of us had a watch, but at some point we opened our eyes and saw a glorious sun setting over a dark, crimson sea. Clouds of varying shades of gray, black, glowing white, and flaming purple filled the sky. They seemed to take the form of giant, flowing letters of fire that didn't really spell anything but communicated a message beyond words.

*Yes!!!!*

Four hours passed like an instant, or perhaps an eternity, and then it started to rain. We had planned to just toss our sleeping bags under the trees down the hill from Highway One, but suddenly the thought of a warm room, a hot shower, and the clean white sheets of a queen-sized bed was irresistible. We drove back up Highway One and took a road east to Salinas. Along the way we told each other what we could about what had just happened. I started telling Julia things about her family and her past that I had no way of knowing. She returned the miracle. At the same time, the intense effects of the acid had passed. I was perfectly capable of driving—even in the pouring rain on a dark, curving coastal highway—although it *did* seem a bit like the car was on automatic pilot.

One strange and wonderful aftereffect persisted into normal consciousness. Somewhere near Salinas, somewhere east of Eden, I slipped my arm around Julia and pulled her toward me. Our skin was no longer a boundary of our separate selves. We melted together every time we touched. That ecstatic feeling continued through that wondrous night. The melting-together feeling continued into the next day, when we felt absolutely sober and straight except when we touched. Back in Berkeley, that feeling—physical and sexual but at the same time spiritual—of melting together every time we touched continued for days, then weeks. There was absolutely no doubt in my eighteen-year-old heart and soul that Julia and I would be together for the rest of our lives. So *this* was love. *This* was what people were talking about when they talked about becoming one with each other. You could *literally* become one with another being. This was bliss. This was ecstasy. This was real.

Or was it?

About a month after the Big Sur trip, Julia and I drove up to the northern end of California with another couple from our Berkeley dorm. We chose this spot at the suggestion of my roommate, whose family were members of a private resort deep in the north woods. It seemed like a great place for a long hike and another trip with that righteous LSD. What my roommate did not mention was that this family resort was actually a hunting lodge with separate dormitories required for unmarried men and women.

LSD's ability to melt the ego and foster a feeling of oneness with the other—with the world—is awesome. It can inspire ecstatic spiritual communion. It can also spark a terrifying existential crisis. Melting into the earth and losing all conception of your skin as the immutable boundary between you and everything else can be wondrous or horrendous—or a simultaneous combination of the two. This second trip in the northern woods was the "bad trip" from central casting. At Big Sur, I'd felt the luscious vastness of the psychedelic experience. But this time around I felt myself shrinking, getting smaller and smaller and terrified of everything around me—including Julia. Suddenly, my soul mate was my adversary. It seemed like she and my two other companions were laughing at me, mocking me. What had been a glimpse into the mind of the mystic became a quick trip into paranoid madness. Of course, it didn't help that we were surrounded by hunting families who were not pleased to see four wacked-out hippies invade their sanctuary, or that we kept hearing gunshots all around us.

Somehow, I managed to make it through the day and back into the dormitory for our second and final night. It was a terrifying, sleepless night, full of voices that may or may not have been imaginary. But what was most frightening was the fact that these paranoid, insecure feelings continued the next morning and on the drive back to Berkeley. Julia was distant, and we soon split up upon our return to campus. She would tell me decades later that she was scared off by my "dark energy."

My confused, paranoid state continued on and off, but mostly on, for weeks. There were frightening LSD flashbacks, but it was more like the drug never really wore off. Chemically, the drug was gone, but psychically and spiritually, the acid trickster would not let me be. I was afraid that I had suffered permanent brain damage. I lost the ability to read—not a good state of mind for a first-year student at the University of California. One word in a sentence would send my mind shooting off on an uncontrollable tangent. There were hallucinations extreme enough that I stopped driving because I couldn't be sure if green lights were really green. Somehow, I succeeded in hiding this insanity from everyone around me. Sharing my state of mind with anyone, I feared, would get me sent to the nearest nuthouse. I stopped taking drugs, including alcohol and marijuana, but it didn't seem to help. I was still stoned out of my mind.

It took a few months, but I somehow got through that hellish descent. The low point came when I was home for the holidays and the hallucinations got so terrifying that I decided to call a mental-health hotline. I ran out to a sidewalk phone booth near my mother's apartment in southern California. When I got into the booth I changed my mind about making the call, only to get trapped inside the glass box—forgetting in my psychotic state that one pulls *inward* to open the accordion doors of those old kiosks. To

the amusement, or perhaps terror, of some passersby, I was franti-
cally pushing out *against* the closed door. Suddenly, I realized what
I was doing. I saw the startled expressions on the faces of the pe-
destrians as I pounded on the door. At the time, I had a bushy
black beard and a long tangle of dark hair, making me look a bit
like Charlie Manson on a bad-hair day. Then I started to laugh.
The joke was on me, but I was able to laugh at myself. To this day,
I recall that hilarious, terrifying moment as the beginning of my
recovery. I pulled open the door of the phone booth and walked
out into the rest of my life.

There would be other battles with drugs and alcohol, but in the
end I think I came out of that teenage experience stronger and
saner than ever. I'd been to the other side, and I'd made it back
alive. It was my version of the hero's journey, but not a trip I recom-
mend for the faint of heart.

Years later, I read a scholarly article by Ralph Metzner, one of
the Harvard graduate students who assisted Timothy Leary and
Richard Alpert in their psychedelic drug research at Harvard. In
the article, titled "Ten Classical Metaphors of Self-Transformation,"
Ralph uses the same symbols I had long used to describe what happened to Julia and me at Big Sur—how our trip began with a return
to "the original state of womb-like unconscious oneness." Metzner
describes the double-edge nature of spiritual growth—especially
when it involves a loss of "skin-bounded ego-consciousness." He
writes, "Whereas for some people the prospect of a transformation
of consciousness is charged with delight, and excitement, for many
the idea of change produces fear."

My two acid trips unfolded in the early 1970s, nearly a decade
after Timothy Leary and Richard Alpert first stressed the importance of the "set and setting" for any psychedelic drug experience.
Make sure you are in a safe, secure, and comfortable place, surrounded by a pleasant environment and people you can trust. In
other words, it's not a good idea for hippies to drop acid at hunting
lodges. At the time, I hadn't heard Leary and Alpert's warning,
and even if I had, I probably would have ignored their advice.

It took me many years to realize that the ecstasy and the agony of my freshman year were not just a great acid trip followed by a bad acid trip. They were the beginning of a long and slow process of spiritual conversion, a painful but ultimately rewarding journey that continues today. Those two psychedelic experiences so long ago left me fascinated with and fearful of the mystical state. They left me curious and skeptical about the spiritual claims of my generation. That curiosity and skepticism led to a long career as a religion writer for the secular press, a perfect perch from which I could "objectively" follow the spiritual journey of my generation of seekers.

Millions of us took LSD and other mind-altering drugs back in the 1960s and 1970s, and many of us are still trying to figure out what it all means. Sometimes I look at the whole spiritual search of my generation—the human-potential movement, the pilgrimages to India, the Buddhist meditation centers, the gurus, the New Age craziness, the "spiritual, but not religious" shift in our attitude toward faith—and I'm convinced that it never would have happened if a Swiss chemist hadn't accidentally dosed himself in a lab mishap at the end of World War II.

Like I said, this book is not about me. It's about four men who can help us figure out what it all means. Was it madness? Was it mysticism? What *did* it all mean? And what does it have to do with the way we lived the rest of our lives? Like many of us, Leary, Alpert, Weil, and Smith were transformed by their psychedelic revelations. Each in his own way discovered how to best bring those powerful experiences into his life. Like us, they stumbled along the way, but in the end, after the ecstasy, they found new meaning and new direction.

So, in the end, perhaps this book is about me. It might also be about you. It's the story of four men whose lives provide a kind of master narrative—a template through which some of us may hear our own stories and, in the process, learn a little something about ourselves.

# ACKNOWLEDGMENTS

It was not my idea alone to write this book. The project began one night in San Francisco over drinks with Mark Tauber, the publisher at HarperOne. We started talking about what I might do to help Huston Smith finish up his long-awaited autobiography. Then Mark had another idea. We continued talking, and you hold the result of that conversation in your hands.

In the introduction, I wrote about the synchronistic coming together of Leary, Alpert, Weil, and Smith. I have the same mysterious feeling about this book. I just told you that my publisher and I met over drinks. That's true, but I was not drinking alcohol. Mark was very surprised at that development. You see, I was not known as someone who'd turn down a free drink—from an editor, publisher, or anyone else. At the time, I'd recently retired from an illustrious, four-decade-long career as a connoisseur of alcohol and other drugs. Use had turned into abuse. I've had a long love/hate affair with drugs, and I hope I have not glorified them too much in this book. That's why I decided to end this book with an acknowledgment of my misadventures with alcohol and other dangerous drugs. So, there you go, dear reader: bottoms up and/or beware.

When I met that night with Mark Tauber, I had just begun a course at the Graduate Theological Union on the psychology of religious conversion, courtesy of a little grant from the Religion Newswriters Association and the Lilly Scholarships in Religion for Journalists. Professor Lewis Rambo had asked his students to begin by writing a "personal conversion narrative." I choose to write about my early experiences with LSD, and I had just started working on that piece of writing when Tauber suggested this book.

Many other people helped me put this work together. They include all those sources who agreed to interviews, but especially Ram Dass, Huston Smith, and Andrew Weil. I would also like to thank Eric Brandt, my editor at HarperOne; Mickey Maudlin, the editorial director at the publishing house; copy editor Carl Walesa and production editor Carolyn Holland. They, along with Amy Rennert, my literary agent, looked over early drafts of the manuscript and made helpful suggestions. The Nieman Foundation for Journalism graciously invited me to a conference that provided a chance to spend some time in Cambridge and conduct a series of interviews at Harvard University and in its environs.

This book would not have been possible without the help of many other people in my supportive circle of family and friends, all of whom have accompanied me on various legs of the long, strange trip. They include my wife, Laura Thomas, along with Janis Crum, Steve Fields, Kevin Griffin, David and Cindy Hoffman, Terry Kupers, Patrick O'Neil, Steve Proctor, Paul and Cheryl Daniels-Shohan, Michael Taylor, Burt Weaver, and the late Maitland "Sandy" Zane.

# BIBLIOGRAPHY

Alpert, Richard [Ram Dass]. *Be Here Now*. San Cristobal, NM: Lama Foundation, 1971.

———. *Grist for the Mill*. Santa Cruz, CA: Unity Press, 1977.

———. Interview by Eliot Jay Rosen. www.vegetarianusa.com/feature_articles/bms/ramdass.html.

———. *Journey of Awakening: A Meditator's Guidebook*. Rev. ed. New York: Bantam, 1990. First published 1978.

———. Letter to Nathan Pusey. *Harvard Crimson*, May 29, 1963.

———. *The Only Dance There Is*. Garden City, NY: Anchor, 1974. First published 1970.

———. "Setisoppoess with Dick Alpert." *San Francisco Oracle*, January 1967, 3.

Alpert, Richard [Ram Dass], and Ralph Metzner, with Gary Bravo. *Birth of a Psychedelic Culture: Conversations About Leary, the Harvard Experiments, Millbrook and the Sixties*. Santa Fe, NM: Synergetic Press, forthcoming.

Alpert, Richard [Ram Dass], with Sidney Cohen and Lawrence Schiller. *LSD*. New York: New American Library, 1966.

Anthony, Gene. *The Summer of Love: Haight-Ashbury at Its Highest*. Oakland, CA: Sixties Foundation, 2002.

Ballard, Paul, ed. *Psychedelic Religion? Papers from a Colloquium*. Cardiff, UK: Collegiate Centre for Theology, University College, 1970.

Bedford, Sybille. *Aldous Huxley: A Biography*. New York: Knopf, 1974.

Bess, Donovan. "Experimenter's Report on Pot and Addiction." *San Francisco Chronicle*, December 14, 1968.

Braden, William. *The Private Sea: LSD and the Search for God*. Chicago: Quadrangle Books, 1967.

Bryan, John. *Whatever Happened to Timothy Leary?* San Francisco: Renaissance Press, 1980.

Chase, Alston. *Harvard and the Unabomber: The Education of an American Terrorist.* New York: W. W. Norton & Company, 2003.

Cheever, Susan. *My Name Is Bill.* New York: Simon & Schuster, 2004.

Cohen, Allen. *The San Francisco Oracle—Facsimile Edition.* Berkeley, CA: Regent Press, 1991.

Clark, Walter Houston. *Chemical Ecstasy: Psychedelic Drugs and Religion.* New York: Sheed and Ward, 1969.

Davidson, Alan. "Holy Man Sighted at Gay Porn House." *Outsmart Magazine,* June 2004.

Doblin, Rick. "Leary's Concord Prison Experiment: A 34-Year Follow-Up Study." *Journal of Psychoactive Drugs* 30, no. 4 (1998): 419–427.

———. "Pahnke's 'Good Friday Experiment': A Long-Term Follow-Up and Methodological Critique." *Journal of Transpersonal Psychology* 23, no. 1 (1991).

Forte, Robert. *Timothy Leary: Outside Looking In.* Rochester, VT: Park Street Press, 1999.

Gates, Barbara, and Wes Nisker. *The Best of Inquiring Mind: 25 Years of Dharma, Drama and Uncommon Insight.* Boston: Wisdom Publications, 2008.

Greenfield, Robert. *Timothy Leary: A Biography.* Orlando, FL: Harcourt, 2006.

Grim, Ryan. *This Is Your Country on Drugs: The Secret History of Getting High in America.* Hoboken, NJ: Wiley, 2009.

Hallgren, Dick. "One Man's Incredible 'Journey.'" *San Francisco Chronicle,* December 19, 1968.

Huxley, Aldous. *The Doors of Perception.* New York: Harper Perennial Library, 2004.

———. *Island.* New York: Harper & Brothers, 1962.

Kilduff, Marshall. "Leary 'Free'—Now to Get Him Out." *San Francisco Chronicle,* June 2, 1973.

Kleps, Art. *Millbrook: The True Story of the Early Years of the Psychedelic Movement.* Portland: Bench Press, 1977.

Kramer, Jane. "Paterfamilias." *New Yorker,* August 17, 1968, 32.

Lattin, Don. "Another Visit to the Oracle." *San Francisco Chronicle,* November 18, 1990.

————. "Chalk It Up to the Counterculture: 60s Survivors Take Some Credit for the World's Social, Political Changes," *San Francisco Chronicle,* February 26, 1990.

————. *Following Our Bliss: How the Spiritual Ideas of the Sixties Shape Our Lives Today.* San Francisco: HarperSanFrancisco, 2003.

————. "Religion Expert Has Had a Long Strange Trip." *San Francisco Chronicle,* January 20, 2002.

————. "Stroke Teaches Ram Dass Anew to 'Be Here Now.'" *San Francisco Chronicle,* May 2, 1997.

————. "Writer Predicts a Return to Hippie Roots." *San Francisco Chronicle,* May 19, 2002.

Leary, Timothy. *Confessions of a Hope Fiend.* New York: Bantam, 1973.

————. *Design for Dying.* New York: HarperEdge, 1997.

————. *Flashbacks: An Autobiography.* Los Angeles: J. P. Tarcher, 1983.

————. *High Priest.* Reprint, Berkeley, CA: Ronin Publishing, 1995.

————. Interview. *Playboy,* September 1966, 93.

————. *Neuropolitique.* Scottsdale, AZ: New Falcon Publications, 1988, 1991.

————. *The Politics of Ecstasy.* Ronin Publishing, 1998. First published 1985 by Grove Press.

————, ed. *The Psychedelic Reader: The Revolutionary 1960s Forum of Psychopharmacological Substances.* New York: Citadel Press, 2007.

Leary, Timothy, with Ralph Metzner and Richard Alpert. *The Psychedelic Experience: A Manual Based on the Tibetan Book of the Dead.* New York: Citadel Press, 2007. First published 1964.

Lee, Martin, and Bruce Shlain. *Acid Dreams: The Complete Social History of LSD: The CIA, the Sixties, and Beyond.* New York: Grove Press, 1985.

Lemley, Brad. "Alternative Medicine Man." *Discover,* August 1999, www.discovermagazine.com/1999/aug/featweil.

MacFarquhar, Larissa. "Andrew Weil, Shaman, M.D." *New York Times Magazine,* August 24, 1997.

Markoff, John. *What the Dormouse Said: How the Sixties Counterculture*

*Shaped the Personal Computer Industry.* New York: Viking Penguin, 2005.

McFague, Sallie. "Conversion: Life on the Edge of the Raft." *Interpretation* 32 (1978): 255–68.

Metzner, Ralph. "Ten Classical Metaphors of Self-Transformation." *Journal of Transpersonal Psychology* 12, no. 1 (1980): 47–62.

Rambo, Lewis R. "Theories of Conversion: Understanding and Interpreting Religious Change." *Social Compass* 46, no. 3 (1999): 259–71.

Rossman, Michael. *New Age Blues: On the Politics of Consciousness.* New York: E. P. Dutton, 1979.

Salinger, J. D. "Teddy." *New Yorker,* January 31, 1953, 26–45.

Slater, Philip. *The Pursuit of Loneliness: American Culture at the Breaking Point.* Boston: Beacon Press, 1970.

Smith, Huston. *Cleansing the Doors of Perception.* New York: Tarcher/Putnam, 2000.

———. *Forgotten Truth.* San Francisco: HarperSanFrancisco, 1992. First published 1976.

———. "The Master-Disciple Relationship." First Victor Danner Memorial Lecture, Indiana University, February 26, 2003.

———. *Why Religion Matters: The Fate of the Human Spirit in an Age of Disbelief.* San Francisco: HarperSanFrancisco, 2001.

———. *The World's Religions.* San Francisco: HarperSanFrancisco, 1991. First published 1958 as *The Religions of Man.*

Smith, Huston, with David Griffin. *Primordial Truth and Postmodern Theology.* Albany, NY: SUNY Press, 1989.

Smith, Huston, with Philip Novak. *Buddhism: A Concise Introduction.* San Francisco: HarperSanFrancisco, 2003.

Smith, Huston, with Jeffrey Paine. *Tales of Wonder: Adventures Chasing the Divine, an Autobiography.* San Francisco: HarperOne, 2009.

Stevens, Jay. *Storming Heaven: LSD and the American Dream.* New York: Harper & Row, 1987.

Taylor, Michael. "How the Swiss React to Leary," *San Francisco Chronicle,* Dec. 26, 1971.

Taylor, Robert. "Baba Ram Dass (the former Richard Alpert, PhD) Shares His Experiences." *Boston Globe Magazine,* June 7, 1970.

Thompson, Mark. *Gay Soul: Finding the Heart of Gay Spirit and Nature.* New York: HarperCollins, 1995.

Ullman, Chana. "Cognitive and Emotional Antecedents of Religious Conversion." *Journal of Personality and Social Psychology* 43, no. 1 (1982): 183–92.

Walsh, Roger, and Charles Grob. *Higher Wisdom: Eminent Elders Explore the Continuing Impact of Psychedelics.* Albany, NY: SUNY Press, 2005.

Watts, Alan. *The Joyous Cosmology.* New York: Pantheon Books, 1962.

Weil, Andrew. *Dr. Andrew Weil's Mindbody Tool Kit Workbook.* Boulder, CO: Sounds True, 2005.

———. *Healthy Aging: A Guide to Your Well-Being.* New York: Anchor Books, 2007.

———. *The Marriage of the Sun and Moon: A Quest for Unity in Consciousness.* Boston: Houghton Mifflin, 1980.

———. *The Natural Mind: A New Way of Looking at Drugs and the Higher Consciousness.* Boston: Houghton Mifflin, 1972.

———. *Spontaneous Healing.* New York: Ballantine Books, 1995.

Weil, Andrew, with Winifred Rosen. *From Chocolate to Morphine: Everything You Need to Know About Mind-Altering Drugs.* Boston: Houghton Mifflin, 1983.

Whitmer, Peter. *Aquarius Revisited: Seven Who Created the Sixties Counterculture That Changed America.* New York: Citadel Press, 1987.

# NOTES ON SOURCE MATERIAL

CHAPTER ONE—FOUR ROADS TO CAMBRIDGE

**Seeker**—This section is drawn from author interviews with Richard Alpert on Maui on January 29–31, 2008, and with Jim Fadiman in Palo Alto, California, on June 18, 2008. Other source material comes from Alpert's *Be Here Now*.

**Trickster**—Drawn from author interviews with Ralph Metzner in San Rafael, California, on February 20, 2008, and with Herbert Kelman, by telephone, on June 18, 2008. Other source material comes from the *San Francisco Chronicle*, October 23, 1955; Leary's autobiography, *Flashbacks;* Robert Greenfield's *Timothy Leary: A Biography;* and Robert Forte's introduction to his *Timothy Leary: Outside Looking In.*

**Healer**—Drawn from author interviews with Andrew Weil in Vail, Arizona, on November 28, 2007, and by telephone on December 4, 2008. Other material comes from *The Natural Mind; Dr. Andrew Weil's Mindbody Tool Kit Workbook; Discover* magazine, August 1999; the *New York Times Magazine,* August 24, 1997; remarks by Weil at a lecture in Oakland, California, on February 9, 2009; and a 1998 Weil interview posted on the Web site of the Academy of Achievement (http://www.achievement.org/autodoc/page/weilint-1).

**Teacher**—Drawn from author interviews with Huston Smith in Berkeley, California, on January 10, 2002, and December 12, 2007, and an interview with Kendra Smith in Berkeley on February 5, 2009. Other source material comes from an early draft of Smith's 2009 autobiography *Tales of Wonder;* Sybille Bedford's *Aldous Huxley: A Biography;* Susan Cheever's *My Name Is Bill;* and Forte.

CHAPTER TWO—TURN ON

**Trickster**—This section is drawn from Leary's accounts in *High Priest* and *Flashbacks*.

**Teacher**—Drawn from author interviews with Smith, along with Huston's account in *Cleansing the Doors of Perception*. Other material comes from Forte's interview with Smith and a tape recording of Humphrey Osmond's account from remarks made at the Esalen Institute in May 1976.

**Seeker**—Drawn from author interviews with Alpert.

**Healer**—Drawn from author interviews with Weil and Alpert, along with an interview with Ronnie Winston conducted in Santa Barbara, California, on March 9, 2008. Some of the Leary quotes at his meeting with Weil and Winston were actually drawn from comments Leary made in a speech before the American Psychological Association on August 30, 1963. Other material comes from Weil's account in *The Natural Mind*.

CHAPTER THREE—SINNERS AND SAINTS

**Trickster**—This section is drawn from author interviews with Metzner and Alpert. Other material comes from Leary's accounts in *Flashbacks;* Osmond's speech at Esalen; Metzner/Alpert conversations in *Birth of a Psychedelic Culture;* and Greenfield and Doblin (1998). The account of Bill Wilson's UCLA trip is from Betty Eisner in Walsh and Grob.

**Teacher**—Drawn from author interviews with Metzner and Smith; with Paul Lee in Santa Cruz on April 9, 2008; and with Harvey Cox in Cambridge on May 10, 2008. Other material comes from Leary's 1983 remarks at Harvard; Smith's account in *Cleansing the Doors of Perception;* and Doblin (1991).

CHAPTER FOUR—CRIMSON TIDE

**Healer**—This section is drawn from author interviews with Kelman, Lee, Weil, and Winston. Other material comes from author interviews with Robert E. Smith in Cambridge, Massachusetts, on May 14, 2008; and with Joe Russin and Bruce Paisner by telephone on May 29,

2008. Alpert's comments at the meeting are partly based on his letter of May 29, 1963.

**Seeker**—Drawn from author interviews with Metzner and Alpert, and from author interview with Peggy Hitchcock by telephone on February 18, 2008. Other material comes from *Birth of a Psychedelic Culture.*

## CHAPTER FIVE—TROUBLE IN PARADISE

**Trickster**—This section is drawn from author interviews with Metzner, Alpert, and Hitchcock. Other material comes from *Flashbacks* and *Birth of a Psychedelic Culture.*

**Seeker**—Drawn from author interviews with Lee, Alpert, and Metzner, and from remarks by Leary and Alpert at Harvard in 1983. Other material comes from *Flashbacks* and John Bryan's *Whatever Happened to Timothy Leary?*

## CHAPTER SIX—IF YOU COME TO SAN FRANCISCO . . .

**Trickster**—Drawn from author interview with Robert Forte in Santa Cruz on June 7, 2008. Other material comes from the *San Francisco Oracle* of January and February 1967; the *San Francisco Chronicle* of May 19, 2002; the *New Yorker* of August 17, 1968; Gene Anthony's book *The Summer of Love;* and *Playboy,* September 1966.

**Seeker**—This section is drawn from author interviews with Alpert and from an author interview with Caroline Winter, via e-mail, on May 26, 2008. Other material comes from Greenfield, Leary's *Neuropolitique,* the *San Francisco Oracle* of January 1967, the *San Francisco Chronicle* of October 29, 1964, and November 3, 1965, and the *Boston Globe Magazine* of June 7, 1970. Additional details came from Jay Stevens's *Storming Heaven* and Martin Lee and Bruce Shlain's *Acid Dreams.*

**Teacher**—Drawn from author interviews with Lee and Smith, and from works cited in text.

**Healer**—Drawn from an author interview with Weil; the *San Francisco Chronicle* of December 19, 1968; *The Natural Mind;* and other works cited in text.

CHAPTER SEVEN—PILGRIMAGE AND EXILE

**Seeker**—This section is based on author interviews with Alpert; with Mirabai Bush in Williamsburg, Massachusetts, on May 13, 2008; and with Wes Nisker in Berkeley, California, on July 7, 2008.

Other material comes from the *San Francisco Chronicle* of May 28, 1968, and March 25, 1973, and the *Boston Globe Magazine* of June 7, 1970. Additional details come from *Be Here Now* and Alpert's remarks at the First Unitarian Church in San Francisco in February 1970 and from his interview in Walsh and Grob.

**Teacher**—Drawn from author interview with Smith. Other material comes from an early draft of Smith's 2009 autobiography; his 2003 book, *Buddhism: A Concise Introduction;* and Smith and David Griffin's book *Primordial Truth and Postmodern Theology.*

**Healer**—Drawn from Weil's accounts in *Spontaneous Healing* and *The Marriage of the Sun and Moon.*

**Trickster**—Drawn from author interviews with Nisker and from author interviews with Brian Barritt, by telephone, on July 18, 2008, and with Dieter Hagenbach, by telephone, on July 11, 2008. Leary's accounts come from *Confessions of a Hope Fiend* and *Flashbacks,* with other details from Bryan and Greenfield.

CHAPTER EIGHT—AFTER THE ECSTASY . . . FOUR LIVES

**Healer**—This section is based on interviews with Weil, and on an interview with his business manager, Richard Baxter, by telephone, on December 15, 2008. Other material comes from *Time* magazine, May 12, 1997; the *New York Times Magazine,* August 24, 1997; and the *New Republic,* December 14, 1998.

**Seeker**—Drawn from author interviews with Alpert and Bush, and from the *San Francisco Chronicle,* July 6, 1991. Other material comes from a 1985 Ram Dass interview in *Inquiring Mind;* his interviews with Mark Thompson, Alan Davidson, and Eliot Jay Rosen; and Michael Rossman's *New Age Blues.*

**Trickster**—Drawn from author interview with Forte. Other material comes from the *San Francisco Chronicle* of June 2, 1973, Greenfield, and Forte.

**Teacher**—Drawn from author interview with Smith. Other material comes from *Tales of Wonder* and *Why Religion Matters*.

Conclusion—Healer, Teacher, Trickster, Seeker

The section on early LSD research in the United States was based on the author's interview with Philip Slater in Santa Cruz on June 8, 2008, along with material from Stevens, Forte, and Lee and Shlain. For more details on the statistics about LSD use in recent decades, see *This Is Your Country on Drugs* by Ryan Grim.

# INDEX

*Page numbers of photos appear in italics.*